Overcoming C̶ ̶ ̶ ̶ ̶ ̶ ̶

Self-d

How to get it and how to keep it

DR WINDY DRYDEN

sheldon **PRESS**

This book is dedicated to the memory of
Jason Krause and Sherrie Myers

First published in Great Britain in 2009

Sheldon Press
36 Causton Street
London SW1P 4ST

Copyright © Dr Windy Dryden 2009

British Library Cataloguing-in-Publication Data
A catalogue record for this book is available from the British Library

ISBN 978–1–84709–086–7

1 3 5 7 9 10 8 6 4 2

Typeset by Fakenham Photosetting Ltd, Fakenham, Norfolk
Printed in Great Britain by Ashford Colour Press

Produced on paper from sustainable forests

Contents

Preface

I have been working as a counsellor in one capacity or another since 1975. In those 30 years or so, I have learned that people could lead far healthier and happier lives if they were more self-disciplined in key areas of their lives. So I have decided to write this book as my contribution to help people learn the skills and beliefs associated with self-discipline.

This book is divided into five parts. In Part 1, I define self-discipline and outline the approach that I will take throughout this book. This approach is called Rational Emotive Behaviour Therapy (REBT), a form of cognitive behaviour therapy (CBT) founded by the late Albert Ellis, a world-famous clinical psychologist, who died in 2007 while this book was being written.

In Part 2, I discuss the importance of goal-setting and self-monitoring of self-undisciplined behaviour, for if you know the extent of the problems and what you want to achieve you will improve the chances of becoming self-disciplined.

In Parts 3 and 4, I discuss the two main forms of self-indiscipline and how you can address them. In Part III, I focus on the type of self-discipline that involves you taking action, and in Part IV, I concentrate on the type of self-discipline that involves you refraining from acting in a self-undisciplined manner.

Finally, in Part 5, I discuss how you can stay self-disciplined once you have initially achieved your self-discipline goals, and in particular show you how you can use other people as a helping resource in this respect, as well as how to respond when other people wittingly or unwittingly try to sabotage your efforts.

I wish you luck in using this book to achieve your own self-discipline goals. If you would like to share your experiences with me, please write to me care of the publisher.

Windy Dryden
London and Eastbourne

Part 1
Introduction

This is a book about an old-fashioned concept that has been neglected but is due for a comeback. No matter how talented you are in life, talent on its own will not get you far. But talent plus self-discipline will. So what is self-discipline? This is the subject for Chapter 1, in which I will consider the concept of self-discipline and break it down into its component parts.

In Chapter 2, I will outline the basic principles of an approach to counselling and psychotherapy known as Rational Emotive Behaviour Therapy (REBT) that I will use throughout this book to help you to become more self-disciplined. REBT is an approach within the tradition of cognitive behaviour therapy (CBT), which has received a lot of favourable press attention as well as proving to be an effective approach to a range of common problems, including where self-indiscipline is a defining characteristic.

1

What is self-discipline?

'What I need is greater self-discipline!' How many times have you heard yourself or other people say something like that? Well, there is good news and bad news!

First, the good news. You *can* learn to become more self-disciplined. This is true even if you think that you are completely self-undisciplined. The bad news is that becoming more self-disciplined is not easy. I wish it was, but generally it is not. Indeed, developing greater self-discipline is something of a paradox, in that you need to be disciplined in order to become more self-disciplined!

But enough of the problems and technicalities. Let's make a start by considering exactly what self-discipline is. I believe that if you know what self-discipline is, then this will help you develop it. So, in this chapter, I will consider the concept of self-discipline and look carefully at its five components.

What is self-discipline?

Having researched the concept of self-discipline in preparation for writing this book, I have concluded that self-discipline has five components:

- *component 1*: improvement
- *component 2*: the 'long-term self' (i.e. the self pursuing improvement)
- *component 3*: obstacles impeding improvement
- *component 4*: the 'short-term self' (i.e. the self engaging with the obstacles)
- *component 5*: the 'executive self' (the self that mediates between the 'long-term self' and the 'short-term self').

Since existing dictionaries (both general and professional) only hint at the five components of self-discipline rather than make them explicit, I decided to come up with my own definition of self-discipline, which appears opposite:

> You are self-disciplined (a) when you have decided to work towards longer-term goals to which you have chosen to commit yourself and to forego shorter-term goals when they are obstacles to achieving these former goals, and (b) when you act on this decision. When you are self-disciplined you acknowledge that there is a part of you that wishes to satisfy the shorter-term goals, but you are able to stand back and choose to pursue what is in your own best interests.

Each of the five components explicitly appears in my definition. Thus:

- Component 1: *Improvement* (my definition mentions 'longer-term goals to which you have chosen to commit yourself').
- Component 2: *Long-term self* (my definition mentions a part of you that has decided to work towards longer-term goals and that takes action in the service of these goals).
- Component 3: *Obstacles* (my definition mentions 'shorter-term goals when they are obstacles to achieving these former [i.e. longer-term] goals'].
- Component 4: *Short-term self* (my definition mentions 'a part of you that wishes to satisfy the shorter-term goals').
- Component 5: *Executive self* (my definition mentions a part of you that is 'able to stand back and choose to pursue what is in your own best interests').

I will now discuss these five components in greater detail.

Improvement

If you consider the concept of improvement, you will see that it is a general term which suggests a state that is healthy or good for you. Broadly speaking, such states enhance your well-being (physical, psychological and, if relevant, spiritual). If you have not already achieved such states then their achievement is usually in the longer term, and generally you have to expend effort and/or deny yourself pleasure to achieve them. For example, if it is healthy for you to weigh 147 lb and you currently weigh 167 lb, then the achievement of the healthy state lies in the future and involves denying yourself pleasure (i.e. you need to refrain from eating high calorie tasty foodstuffs) and expending effort (if exercise plays a part in your weight loss programme).

Who defines your goals?

You will increase the chances of being self-disciplined if you define for yourself what is healthy or good for you. If others define this and you disagree with them, then your motivation to pursue this so-called 'healthy' or 'good' state will be quite low. Indeed, if you are what psychologists call 'reactant' (meaning highly sensitive to having your sense of autonomy threatened), then you will not pursue this state precisely *because* others have defined it as productive for you, even if you agree with them.

However, even if you do decide what is healthy or good for you, this is not, on its own, sufficient to promote self-discipline.

Make a commitment to seek improvement

How many times have you heard someone say something like 'I know I should get down to work …'? Probably many times. And you have probably said something like that yourself, again many times. What a statement like this signifies is that you know what is good for you but you don't act on it. What is missing here is making a commitment to pursue whatever it is you have defined as being healthy for you. Committing yourself to a sustained course of healthy action is important in that when you make such a commitment, you decide to act on what you know is healthy. Without such a commitment all you have is an acknowledgment that a course of action is healthy, and this acknowledgment on its own very often does not lead to self-discipline.

Making a commitment to take a particular course of healthy action is important when you are faced with a number of such courses of action but are unable or unwilling to follow all of them. In committing to a particular course of healthy action, you are choosing among the available courses of action on offer and deciding to implement one.

Take action

While making a commitment to follow a course of action is important, it is insufficient to achieve your goals. Taking action is the only reliable way to achieve improvement. A commitment is a cognitive or thinking procedure, while taking action involves behaviour and it is only behaviour that will enable you to achieve your longer-term goals.

Let me illustrate what I mean by discussing the writing of this book. For quite a while now I have wanted to write a book on self-discipline, but I have had a number of other projects. Once I had completed these projects I made a commitment to write this book. However, I had to act on this commitment and actually write at least 500 words a day (my writing regime involves writing 500 words every day) in order to achieve my goal. This is what I did, and you are reading the results of my decision to act on my commitment to write this book.

When you choose not to take action in the service of your goals, but rather choose to take some other action, it is important that you understand the factors in operation at that time. It may be that you find the goal-related action uncomfortable, anxiety-provoking or anger-engendering, to give three examples. Whatever the reason, you need to identify those factors and deal with them effectively, otherwise you will not achieve your self-discipline goals.

Achievement vs. maintenance

While achieving your self-discipline goals is important, this is only half the story. Thus, in the earlier example, where you had to lose 20 lb for health reasons, it is one thing to achieve the weight target of 147 lb but it is quite another to maintain it. In general, while the achievement of any long-term goal that involves effort and/or restraint is difficult, it is much harder to maintain such gains. To do so, you need to make enduring changes in your behavioural repertoire. Let's assume that you altered your eating behaviour and lost 20 lb, but once you did so you immediately went back to your previous high calorie diet. What would happen? Quite clearly you would put on the weight that you lost, and in all probability more quickly than it took you to lose it in the first place. So if you wanted to maintain your weight at 147 lb, you would have to make enduring changes to your eating habits, and deal effectively with threats to ongoing self-disciplined behaviour.

Long-term self

What I have called the long-term self (LTS) is the part of you entrusted with the task of looking after your long-term healthy interests from a psychological, physical and, if relevant, spiritual perspective. When fulfilling this task, the long-term self is ever mindful of the longer term rather than the shorter term. Your LTS is the part of you that reminds you 'no gains without pains' and 'if you want something, then you have to work for it'. This part of you encourages you to make short-term sacrifices for long-term gains. Thus, it urges you to refrain from behaviours that are pleasurable, but self-defeating in the longer term. It reminds you of your healthy long-term goals and that the effort to achieve them is worth it.

Again, when doing its job correctly, your LTS shows you that you, as a person, are worth making sacrifices for. It is therefore also concerned with encouraging you to develop, maintain and act on a healthy attitude towards yourself.

Obstacles

You can engage with many things which serve as obstacles to self-discipline in the sense that this engagement interferes with you pursuing your long-term goals. These things tend to be pleasurable or less aversive than the activities that would lead to goal achievement. Here are a couple of examples:

- Gerry was in the final year of his degree. He had planned to work on an essay on Thursday evening, but when one of his friends dropped by unexpectedly and asked him to go out to a party, Gerry agreed to go and left with his work undone.
- Laurence was on the same course as Gerry and planned to work on the same essay that Thursday night. But instead of getting down to work, he spent the evening tidying his study in preparation for working on the essay.

In Gerry's case, he was faced with a choice between working on his essay, which he found boring, or going to a party, a prospect that he found exciting. He chose to go to the party. At this point the party became an obstacle. Before Gerry made that decision, going to the party was a potential obstacle.

In Laurence's case, he was faced with a choice between working on his essay, which he found anxiety-provoking, and tidying his room, which he found boring but which reduced his anxiety. When Laurence chose to involve himself in tidying his study, this activity became an obstacle for him. Before he did so, it again was a potential obstacle.

Short-term self

The short-term self (STS) is concerned with satisfying your basic instincts. It is not at all concerned with your longer-term healthy interests. Its motto might be said to be 'Eat, drink and be merry, for tomorrow you might die.' As such, it is the part of you that is your own biggest block to developing self-discipline. The STS is not only concerned with pleasure, it is also concerned with the relief of pain and discomfort in their broadest sense.

Fortunately, it is rare that a person is completely dominated by his or her STS, but when this happens it has catastrophic results. Many years ago, I attended a case conference in Manhattan. The person we were considering was a 32-year-old man who had inherited vast wealth. He was obese, very unfit and spent a considerable amount of money each week paying people to do basic chores for him: cleaning his apartment, making his food, washing him and even cleaning his teeth! The question we were asked to address in the case conference was: should the therapist who was being asked to take on this person as a client go to his apartment to carry out therapy or not, given that the client would not come to the therapist's office? The person was miserable, but wouldn't do anything to help himself because he was dominated by his STS.

Executive self

This fifth and final component of self-discipline is what I call the executive self (ES). This is the part of you that mediates between your long-term and short-term selves. It helps to ensure that you have a healthy balance in life between pursuing your longer-term goals and satisfying your shorter-term goals. This dispels a common misconception that the major task of the executive self is to ensure that the long-term self is in control. If this were the case then you would only be pursuing your longer-term goals and you would have no short-term fun. This would be like putting your money in a savings account and never spending any of it.

On the other hand, if your STS were in the driving seat then this would be like spending everything you had (and probably getting into debt!) and saving nothing. The task of the executive self is to make sure that you make an investment in your future and that you pursue short-term enjoyment too – in other words, that you live a balanced life rather than one of either austerity or profligacy. As we will see, your ES is at its most efficient when it helps you to attend to your long-term self before attending to your short-term self, rather than vice versa, although exceptions to this 'rule' are permitted!

● Simon was on the same course as Gerry and Laurence, whom I discussed above, and had the same essay to do. When Gerry and his friend knocked on his door to invite him to the party, Simon declined, saying that he was going to finish the essay that night and then go out to the pub the next night to let his hair down.

Having introduced the concept of self-discipline and briefly discussed its five basic components, in the next chapter I will consider the long-term self in greater detail and show how to get the most out of it.

2

The REBT model

Any approach to self-discipline is based on a set of assumptions concerning the factors that explain both self-discipline and self-indiscipline. This book is based on an approach to counselling and psychotherapy called Rational Emotive Behaviour Therapy (REBT), created and developed by the famous American clinical psychologist Dr Albert Ellis. As I have said, REBT is an approach within the cognitive behavioural therapeutic tradition (CBT). The basic idea of CBT can be summed up in the famous dictum attributed to the Greek philosopher Epictetus (*c.* 55–*c.* 135 CE):

> People are disturbed not by things, but by their views of things.

The basic idea of REBT can be summed up in the following modification to Epictetus' dictum:

> People are disturbed not by things, but by their rigid and extreme views of things.

If we apply the REBT dictum to self-discipline, we have the following:

> People act in a self-undisciplined manner when they hold rigid and extreme views about threats to self-discipline.

Holding these rigid and extreme views about such threats to self-discipline leads people to attempt to eliminate the threats as quickly as they can. This usually involves acting in a self-undisciplined way. Thus, if you feel an urge to smoke a cigarette when you are attempting to refrain from smoking and you hold rigid and extreme views about this urge, then you will tend to smoke the cigarette (or engage in some other self-undisciplined behaviour) in order to eliminate the urge.

REBT's situational ABC model

REBT puts forward a straightforward 'situational ABC' model of self-discipline and self-indiscipline, and this is the best way of understanding REBT's contribution to this topic. So let me outline this model in its basic form before discussing each element in greater detail.

'Situation'

You do not react in a vacuum. Rather, you think, feel and act in specific situations. The 'situation' in the ABC refers to a descriptive account of the actual event to which you respond with self-discipline or self-indiscipline.

'A' = activating event

Within this specific situation, when you respond in a self-disciplined or self-undisciplined manner, it is usually to a key aspect of this situation. This is known as an activating event (or 'A').

'B' = belief

It is a major premise of REBT that while your emotions and behaviour are usually in response to an activating event or 'A', the 'A' does not cause this emotional/behavioural reaction. Rather, your emotions and behaviour are primarily determined by the beliefs that you hold about the 'A'.

'C' = the three consequences of the beliefs at 'B' about the activating event at 'A'

When you hold a belief about an 'A', you will tend to (1) experience an emotion, (2) act in a certain way and (3) think in certain ways. These three consequences of this 'A' × 'B' interaction are known as emotional, behavioural and thinking consequences, respectively.

Let me now discuss each of these elements in greater detail.

'Situation'

As I said earlier, self-disciplined or self-undisciplined episodes do not take place in a vacuum. Rather, they occur in specific 'situations'. Such 'situations' are viewed in the situational ABC model as descriptions of actual events about which you form inferences (see below). 'Situations' exist in time. Thus, they can describe past actual events (e.g. 'My boss offered me a cigarette'), present actual events (e.g. 'My boss is offering me a cigarette') or future events (e.g. 'My boss will offer me a cigarette when we go out for a drink at the end of the day'). Note that I have not referred to such future events as future actual events, since you don't know that such events will occur and such future events may prove to be false. But if you look at such future 'situations', they are still descriptions of what may happen and do not add inferential meaning (see below).

'Situations' may refer to internal actual events (i.e. events that occur within yourself, e.g. thoughts, feelings, bodily sensations, aches and pains, etc.) or to external actual events (i.e. events that occur outside yourself, e.g. your boss asking to see you). Their defining characteristic is as before: they are descriptions of events and do not include inferential meaning.

'A'

'A', an activating event, is the aspect of the situation about which you respond with self-discipline or self-indiscipline. Let me make a number of points about 'A'.

An 'A' is usually an inference and needs to be differentiated from the 'situation' or actual event about which it is made

An inference is basically an interpretation or hunch about the 'situation', whereas the 'situation' is purely descriptive. Let me provide you with an example to make this distinction clear.

Imagine that your boss asks you out for a drink at the end of the day. You think that this means that she is going to offer you a cigarette at a time when you have just given up smoking and that if she does you will be tempted to accept the offer. The situation or actual event is: 'My boss has asked me out for a drink at the end of the day', while your 'A' is: 'My boss is going to offer me a cigarette and I will accept.' As can be seen from this example, the 'situation' is a description of the facts of the matter whereas the 'A' is a key inference that you have made about the 'situation'. It is key because it is the aspect of the situation to which you have an emotional response (in this case anxiety). When you have a significant emotional response to an event or 'situation', the 'A' represents the personalized inferential meaning that you give to the situation.

Inferences that usually comprise the 'A' can be true or false and, as such, when you make an inference you need to evaluate it against the available evidence

Thus, in our example, it may be true or false that your boss will offer you a cigarette when you both go out for a drink. Also, if she does, it may be true or false that you will be tempted to accept the offer. All you can do is to consider the available evidence and come up with the 'best bet' about what is going to happen at drinks with your boss. This involves considering such factors as: (1) what has happened in the past when your boss has taken you out for drinks; and (2) what has happened in the past when people have offered you a cigarette when you were trying to 'kick the habit'.

An 'A' can be about an event external to you or about an event internal to you

The defining characteristic of this 'A' is again its inferential nature. For example:

External 'situation' = Friend asks me to go to the pub
'A' about external 'situation' = He wants to stop me from working on my essay
Internal 'situation' = A feeling of anxiety
'A' about internal 'situation' = I am losing control

'B'

Beliefs are attitudes which can be rational (or healthy) or irrational (or unhealthy). You can hold beliefs about descriptive 'situations', but more often you will hold beliefs about the inferences at 'A' that you make about these more objective 'situations'.

Rational beliefs

REBT argues that rational beliefs have five major characteristics. They are:

1 flexible or non-extreme;
2 conducive to your mental health;
3 helpful to you as you strive towards your goals;
4 true;
5 logical.

REBT theory puts forward four rational beliefs.

Non-dogmatic preference

Human beings have desires, and for desires to be the cornerstone of healthy functioning they take the form of non-dogmatic preferences. A non-dogmatic preference has two components:

- *An 'asserted preference' component*: here, you make clear to yourself what you want (either what you want to happen or exist or what you want not to happen or exist).
- *A 'negated demand' component*: here you acknowledge that what you want to occur or exist does not have to occur or exist.

In short, we have:

> Non-dogmatic preference = 'asserted preference' component + 'negated demand' component

Thus, if your boss offered you a cigarette your non-dogmatic preference would be: 'I want to have a cigarette, but I don't have to have one.' This belief would help you to say 'no' to the cigarette and thus act in a self-disciplined manner.

Non-awfulizing belief

When your non-dogmatic preference is not met, it is healthy for you to conclude that it is bad that you have not got what you wanted. It is not healthy to be indifferent about not getting what you desire. As with a non-dogmatic preference, a non-awfulizing belief has two components.

- An *'asserted badness'* component: here, you acknowledge that it is bad that you have not got what you want or that you have got what you don't want.
- A *'negated awfulizing'* component: here, you acknowledge that while it is bad when you don't get your desires met, it is not awful, terrible or the end of the world.

In short, we have:

> Non-awfulizing belief = 'asserted badness' component + 'negated awfulizing' component

Thus, if your boss offered you a cigarette your non-awfulizing belief would be: 'It is bad not having a cigarette, but it isn't terrible not having one.' This belief would also help you to say 'no' to the cigarette and thus act in a self-disciplined manner.

High frustration tolerance (HFT) belief

When your non-dogmatic preference is not met it is healthy for you to conclude that it is difficult for you to tolerate not getting what you want, but that you can tolerate it. An HFT belief has three components.

- An *'asserted struggle'* component: here, you recognize that it is a struggle to put up with not getting what you want.
- A *'negated unbearability'* component: here, you acknowledge that while it is a struggle to tolerate not getting your desires met, it is not intolerable.
- A *'worth tolerating'* component: this points to the fact that not only can you tolerate not getting what you want, but that it is worth it to you to do so.

In short, we have:

> High frustration tolerance belief = 'asserted struggle' component + 'negated unbearability' component + 'worth tolerating' component

Thus, if your boss offered you a cigarette your HFT belief would be: 'It is a struggle not having a cigarette, but I can tolerate the struggle and it is worth it to me to do so.' This belief would again help you to say 'no' to the cigarette and thus act in a self-disciplined manner.

Acceptance belief

When your non-dogmatic preference is not met it is healthy for you to accept this state of affairs. There are three types of acceptance belief:

1 a self-acceptance belief where you accept yourself for not meeting your desires or for not having them met;
2 an other-acceptance belief where you accept another person or other people for not meeting your desires; and
3 an acceptance of life conditions belief where you accept life conditions when they don't meet your desires.

There are three components to an acceptance belief, which I will illustrate with reference to a self-acceptance belief.

1 A *'negatively evaluated aspect' component*: here, you recognize when you have not met your desires or that your desires have not been met by others or by life conditions, and you evaluate this particular aspect negatively.
2 A *'negated global negative evaluation' component*: here, you acknowledge that while you may have acted badly, for example, or experienced a bad event, the whole of you is not bad.
3 An *'asserted complex and/or fallibility' component*: here, you assert that you are a complex fallible human being for acting badly.

In short, we have:

Acceptance belief = 'negatively evaluated aspect' component + 'negated global negative evaluation' component + 'asserted complexity and/or fallibility' component

Thus, if your boss offered you a cigarette your acceptance of life conditions belief (in this case) would be: 'It is bad not having a cigarette, but life isn't all bad when I don't have one. It's a mixture of good, bad and neutral things.' Yet again, this belief would help you to say 'no' to the cigarette and thus act in a self-disciplined manner.

Irrational beliefs

REBT argues that irrational beliefs have five major characteristics. They are:

1 rigid or extreme

2 conducive to psychological disturbance
3 unhelpful to you as you strive towards your goals
4 false
5 illogical.

REBT theory puts forward four irrational beliefs.

Demand

REBT theory holds that when you take your desires and turn them into rigid demands, absolute necessities, musts, absolute shoulds and the like, you make yourself disturbed when you don't get what you believe you must. Even when you do get what you believe you must, you are still vulnerable to disturbance when you hold a rigid demand at the point when you become aware that you might lose what you have and need.

A rigid demand has two components.

- An 'asserted preference' component: this is the same as the 'asserted preference' component of a non-dogmatic preference. Again, you make clear to yourself what you want (either what you want to happen or exist or what you want not to happen or exist).
- An 'asserted demand' component: here you take what you want and you turn it into a 'rigid demand' (e.g. 'I want to have a cigarette and therefore I have to have one').

In short, we have:

> Rigid demand = 'asserted preference' component + 'asserted demand' component

Thus, if your boss offered you a cigarette your demand, as shown above, would be: 'I want to have a cigarette and therefore I must have one.' This belief would lead you to take the cigarette and thus act in a self-undisciplined manner.

Awfulizing belief

When your rigid demand is not met then you will tend to make the extreme conclusion that it is awful, horrible, terrible or the end of the world that you haven't got what you insist you must have. As with a non-awfulizing belief, an awfulizing belief has two components.

- An 'asserted badness' component: this component is the same as that in the non-awfulizing belief. Here you acknowledge that it is bad that you have not got what you want or that you have got what you don't want.
- An 'asserted awfulizing' component: here, you take your non-extreme

evaluation of badness and transform it into an extreme evaluation of horror (e.g. 'Because it would be bad if I were to deprive myself of a cigarette, it would be horrible were I to do so').

In short, we have:

> Awfulizing belief = 'asserted badness' component + 'asserted awfulizing' component

Thus, if your boss offered you a cigarette, your awfulizing belief would be: 'It is not only bad not having a cigarette, it is terrible not to have one.' This belief would also lead you to take the cigarette and thus act in a self-undisciplined manner.

Low frustration tolerance (LFT) belief

When your rigid demand is not met, you will tend to make the extreme conclusion that you can't bear not getting what you demand. Unlike an HFT belief, which has three components, an LFT belief tends to have only two components.

- *An 'asserted struggle' component*: as with your HFT belief, here you recognize that it is a struggle to put up with not getting what you want.
- *An 'asserted unbearability' component*: here, you acknowledge that it is not just a struggle to put up with not getting your demand met, it is intolerable. Since you think that you cannot put up with not getting your demand met, the issue of whether or not it is worth tolerating does not arise. You can't tolerate it and that's that.

In short, we have:

> Low frustration tolerance belief = 'asserted struggle' component + 'asserted unbearability' component

Thus, if your boss offered you a cigarette your LFT belief would be: 'It's a struggle not having a cigarette and I can't bear this struggle.' This belief would again lead you to take the cigarette and thus act in a self-undisciplined manner.

Depreciation belief

When your rigid demands are not met you will tend to depreciate yourself, depreciate others or depreciate life conditions. Thus, there are three types of depreciation belief:

1 a self-depreciation belief where you depreciate yourself for not meeting your demands or for not having them met;

2 an other-depreciation belief where you depreciate another person or other people for not meeting your demands; and
3 a depreciation of life conditions belief where you depreciate life conditions when they don't meet your demands.

There are two components to a depreciation belief, which I will illustrate with reference to a self-depreciation belief.

• A *'negatively evaluated aspect' component*: here, you recognize that you have not met your demands or that your demands have not been met by others or by life conditions and, as in the corresponding acceptance belief, you evaluate this particular aspect negatively.
• An *'asserted global negative evaluation' component*: here, you give yourself a global negative rating for not meeting your demands (or for not having your demands met). Thus, you may acknowledge that you have acted badly as you believe you absolutely should not have done, and then evaluate yourself as a bad person for acting badly.

In short, we have:

> Depreciation belief = 'negatively evaluated aspect' component + 'asserted global negative evaluation' component

Thus, if your boss offered you a cigarette your life-depreciation belief would be: 'It is bad not having a cigarette and therefore life is all bad when I don't have one.' Yet again, this belief would encourage you to take the cigarette and thus act in a self-undisciplined manner.

'C'

'C' stands for the consequences that you experience when you hold a belief at 'B' about 'A'. There are three major consequences, which I will consider separately but which in reality occur together.

Emotional 'C's

When your 'A' is negative and you hold a set of rational beliefs at 'B' about this 'A', your emotional 'C' will be negative but healthy. Yes, that's right: negative emotions can be healthy. Thus, when you face a threat it is healthy to feel concerned, and when you have experienced a loss it is healthy to feel sad. Other healthy negative emotions (so called because they feel unpleasant but help you to deal constructively with negative life events) are: remorse, disappointment, sorrow, healthy anger, healthy jealousy and healthy envy.

When your 'A' is negative, but this time you hold a set of irrational beliefs at 'B' about this 'A', your emotional 'C' will be negative and unhealthy. Thus, when you face a threat it is unhealthy to feel anxious, and when you have experienced a loss it is unhealthy to feel depressed. Other unhealthy negative emotions (so called because they feel unpleasant and they interfere with you dealing constructively with negative life events) are: guilt, shame, hurt, unhealthy anger, unhealthy jealousy and unhealthy envy.

There are occasions when people act in self-disciplined ways to cope with these unhealthy negative emotions, and when this occurs it is important to target these emotions for change as a way of promoting self-disciplined behaviour.

Behavioural 'C's

When your 'A' is negative and you hold a set of rational beliefs at 'B' about this 'A', your behavioural 'C' is likely to be constructive. Such behaviour is constructive in three ways. First, it will help you to change the negative event that you are facing if it can be changed. Second, it will help you to make a healthy adjustment if the event cannot be changed; and third, it will help you to go forward and make progress at achieving your goals. This is particularly relevant for our discussion of self-discipline.

When your 'A' is negative, but this time you hold a set of irrational beliefs at 'B' about this 'A', your behavioural 'C' will be unconstructive. Such behaviour is unconstructive in three ways. First, it won't help you to change the negative event that you are facing if it can be changed. Indeed, such unconstructive behaviour will often make a bad situation worse. Second, it will prevent you from making a healthy adjustment if the event cannot be changed; and third, it will take you away from pursuing your goals and make you prone to self-undisciplined behaviour.

Thinking 'C's

When your 'A' is negative and you hold a set of rational beliefs at 'B' about this 'A', your subsequent thinking (or thinking 'C') is likely to be constructive. Such thinking is constructive in two ways.

- It is realistic and allows you to deal with probable outcomes.
- It is balanced and recognizes, for example, that you will get a range of positive, neutral and negative responses to your behaviour.

As a result, these thinking 'C's enable you to respond constructively to realistically perceived situations and help protect you from acting in self-undisciplined ways.

When your 'A' is negative, but this time you hold a set of irrational beliefs at 'B' about this 'A', your subsequent thinking (or thinking 'C') is likely to be unconstructive. Such thinking is unconstructive in two ways.

- It is unrealistic in that you will tend to think that low probability, highly aversive outcomes are far more likely to happen than the data suggest.
- It is skewed in that you think that the consequences of your negative behaviour will be entirely negative. In reality, such consequences are likely to be mixed: some negative, some neutral and even some positive.

As a result, these thinking 'C's interfere with your ability to respond constructively to realistically perceived situations and make you more prone to self-undisciplined behaviour.

Summary

Let me summarize what I have discussed in this chapter in diagrammatic form. Table 1 summarizes REBT's position on rational and irrational beliefs at 'B' in the situational ABC model.

Table 1 Irrational and rational beliefs in REBT theory

Irrational belief	Rational belief
Demand X must (or must not) happen	Non-dogmatic preference I would like X to happen (or not happen), but it does not have to be the way I want it to be
Awfulizing belief It would be terrible if X happens (or does not happen)	Non-awfulizing belief It would be bad, but not terrible, if X happens (or does not happen)
LFT belief I could not bear it if X happens (or does not happen)	HFT belief It would be difficult to bear if X happens (or does not happen), but I could bear it and it would be worth it to me to do so
Depreciation belief If X happens (or does not happen) I am no good/you are no good/life is no good	Acceptance belief If X happens (or does not happen), it does not prove that I am no good/you are no good/life is no good. Rather, I am an FHB/you are an FHB/life is a complex mixture of good, bad and neutral

FHB = Fallible human being
LFT = Low frustration tolerance
HFT = High frustration tolerance

Table 2 outlines the situational ABC model where your beliefs are rational.

Table 2 Situational ABC model where your beliefs are rational

Situation	Objectively described event
Negative 'A'	Aspect of the situation to which you respond emotionally, behaviourally and cognitively
'B' (rational belief)	Non-dogmatic preference Non-awfulizing belief High frustration tolerance belief Acceptance belief
'C' (consequences)	Emotional (healthy negative) Behavioural (constructive) Thinking (realistic and balanced)

Table 3 outlines the situational ABC model where your beliefs are irrational.

Table 3 Situational ABC model where your beliefs are irrational

Situation	Objectively described event
Negative 'A'	Aspect of the situation to which you respond emotionally, behaviourally and cognitively
'B' (irrational belief)	Demand Awfulizing belief Low frustration tolerance belief Depreciation belief
'C' (consequences)	Emotional (unhealthy negative) Behavioural (unconstructive) Thinking (unrealistic and skewed)

Hopefully, the REBT model makes sense to you and you can see how it can help you to become more self-disciplined. If so, proceed to the next part of the book, where I will discuss how you can get the best out of your long-term self.

Part 2

Get the most out of your long-term self

As I said in the opening chapter, when we consider the concept of self-discipline three different parts of you come into play. I call these (1) the long-term self, (2) the short-term self and (3) the executive self. In this part of the book, I will concentrate on the long-term self (henceforth known as the LTS).

Your LTS is charged with the task of looking after your healthy long-term interests, and its communications to you will be all about this aspect of your life. Without your LTS you would live a life of pleasure and hedonism, free from the irksome responsibilities of life. Does this sound attractive? Yes? But wait a moment: to achieve this, you would probably have to be independently wealthy and pay someone to do all your chores and basically deal with the uncomfortable aspects of life for you. Does this apply to you? Even if it does and you manage all of this, would you really be happy? You might think so, but actually you wouldn't be. Studies of happiness have shown that we are at our happiest when we are actively working on projects that are personally meaningful to us. Such active work usually involves effort, which is often uncomfortable, at least at the beginning.

You will also need to pay attention to your LTS if your physical health is important to you. It is one of life's frustrations that often the things that are pleasurable are bad for us in the long term. Take food, for example. Most foods that taste good, either sweet or savoury, are not good for us if we eat them to excess. A survey of women's favourite foods in America found that the top three favourite foods were: (1) chocolate, (2) chocolate (cake) and (3) chocolate (ice cream). Note that it wasn't broccoli, carrots and spinach! So if you are going to live healthily, then you will need to access and listen to your LTS. Even more importantly, you need to act on its promptings.

3

Set goals for self-discipline

The first step that you need to take in your quest for greater self-discipline in your life is to set goals for self-discipline. As I will show you in a minute, this involves you asking yourself and answering two fundamental questions:

- Is it worth doing?
- Am I worth doing it for?

Before you address these two questions, I want to stress that the best way of setting goals for self-discipline is within a context of balanced living, and it is to this issue that I will now turn.

Set goals for self-discipline within the context of balanced living

As I discussed in Chapter 1, you have three parts of you that are relevant to the enterprise of developing self-discipline: your short-term self (STS), your long-term self (LTS) and your executive self (ES). When you come to set goals which require self-discipline, you will increase your chance of success if you embed these goals within the context of balanced living.

Ensure that you have some pleasure in your life

By 'balanced living', I mean looking after yourself and your healthy interests (in the short and longer term) while ensuring that some of your short-term hedonistic goals are being catered for. So don't set self-discipline goals without ensuring that you have some pleasure in your life. If you do this, the chances are that you will fail in being self-disciplined because you have nothing to look forward to in the short term.

Now, when you do pursue hedonistic pleasure in the short term, it is often important that this is in a different area from the area that you are going to set goals. So if you have set refraining from smoking as a self-discipline goal, then it is best not to seek short-term pleasure from smoking. However, if you are working to eat healthily it is probably sensible not to exclude all fattening foods from your diet. Satisfying some of these desires will help you develop a balanced diet rather than an austere one. Having said this, if having one square of chocolate means that you have to have three bars, then it is best not to have the one square until you have developed a greater sense of control and have challenged the all-or-nothing thinking which lies behind the lack of self-control.

It is the task of your ES to negotiate between your STS and your LTS. In accessing your ES, you need to be particularly aware that your STS is good at seducing you into pursuing the pleasure of the moment under the guise of balanced living. If you are mindful of this and question yourself quite closely, you will be less likely to be seduced into pursuing short-term goals which interfere with self-discipline. Rather, you will allow yourself short-term pleasure, but only after you have acted in a self-disciplined manner. Here, you make engaging in pleasure conditional on first acting in a self-disciplined way.

Pursue meaning in life

It is probably easier for you to engage in self-disciplined activities if you are also actively pursuing meaningful life goals. These goals will help to sustain you when the going gets tough, as it almost certainly will as you strive to be more self-disciplined. Although these meaningful goals may not be directly relevant to your self-discipline goals, they can frequently serve as potent forms of motivation to stay on track. For example, Kerry went on a healthy diet but struggled in dealing with her inner urges to eat tasty but fattening foods. A year later she tried again to develop and maintain healthy eating habits. In the time between the two episodes, Kerry became involved in starting and running a children's book club because she passionately felt that children would benefit from reading novels, short stories and poetry. Having involved herself in this meaningful pursuit, Kerry was more successful in dealing with her urges to eat fattening foods, for two main reasons. First, she reminded herself (1) that she did not need to eat these foods to make her life meaningful (which she had believed before) and (2) that her book-club activity, not food, was a reference point for meaning. Second, having dealt with her urges in this way, she *actively* involved herself in some book-club related pursuits, thus *putting into practice* the idea that meaning comes from activity and not from food. Learn this lesson from Kerry and involve yourself in meaningful activity which will help you to pursue self-discipline goals. Here, just thinking about meaningful activity will not help you in this respect. Engaging in this activity usually will.

Having made the point that setting goals for self-discipline doesn't preclude you from having short-term pleasure and is best done when you are pursuing meaning in life, let us move on to the topic of setting such goals by first addressing the 'is it worth it?' question.

Is it worth doing?

Perhaps the major task that your LTS has is to help you focus on and identify your healthy long-term goals. Since your LTS knows your interests and values, it can help you to set goals that are really what you want (rather than what others think you should want) and that are based on these interests and values.

Write down your answers to the following questions set by your LTS. Do so on a separate sheet of paper for each area of your life that you select – this is important! If you put all the areas on one sheet, it may well prove too complex and confusing for you and you may be put off before you start.

1 In which area of my life do I want to be more disciplined?
2 Do I really want to be disciplined in this area, or am I only saying so to please others or get them 'off my back'?
3 Why do I want to be disciplined in this area?
4 Which values underpin my reasons and how important are these values in my life, on a scale from 0 = no importance to 10 = very great importance?
5 How committed am I to working to develop and maintain self-discipline in this area, on a scale from 0 = no commitment to 10 = full commitment?

You might find it helpful to use the blank form in Appendix 1. Again, use one form for each life area.

If you find answering these questions difficult, imagine that they are being answered on your behalf by someone who deeply cares about you and wants you to lead an effective life. This person should be someone who knows you deeply and is ruthlessly honest with you.

Let me give you three examples of people who answered the above questions, and let's consider the issues that their responses raise.

Harry's example

1 In which area of my life do I want to be more disciplined?
   I want to stop procrastinating and do tasks when it is in my best interests to do them.
2 Do I really want to be disciplined in this area or am I only saying so to please others or get them 'off my back'?
   I want to do this for myself.
3 Why do I want to be disciplined in this area?
   It would make my life less disorganized and I would feel more in control.
4 Which values underpin my reasons and how important are these values in my life, on a scale from 0 = no importance to 10 = great importance?

Self-control = 9
Organization = 5
Being a good role model for my colleagues = 2
Being a good role model for my kids = 9

5 How committed am I to working to develop and maintain self-discipline in this area, on a scale from 0 = no commitment to 10 = full commitment?
Commitment = 7

Harry's example discussed   The area of self-discipline that Harry has selected (i.e. overcoming procrastination) is notoriously difficult to develop and maintain. Consequently, he needs a high level of commitment and this level needs to be underpinned by important values that will serve to sustain Harry when the going gets tough, which it almost certainly will.

Harry has indicated that he wishes to stop procrastinating and to start doing tasks when it is healthy for him to do so. This is fine as a general statement of goals and he has clearly indicated that he wishes to do this for himself. This is a good sign since Harry is self-motivated.

Harry then lists four values that underpin his self-discipline goals: two which are strong ('self-control', '9', and 'being a good role model for my kids', '9'), one which is medium ('organization', '5') and one which is weak ('being a good role model for my work colleagues', '2'). Generally speaking, the greater the number of strong values that underpin your self-discipline goals, the greater the chance you have of doing what you need to do to achieve these goals.

Finally, Harry's stated level of commitment is reasonably high ('7') and consistent with his value ratings. Sometimes, people may say that they are very committed to achieving a self-discipline goal but this is not consistent with the strength of their value ratings (see Barbara's example, below). In this case, the person needs to identify and address reasons for this inconsistency. Normally, it is because the person has exaggerated his or her level of commitment – a common situation which is predictive of self-discipline failure.

Sandra's example

1 In which area of my life do I want to be more disciplined?
I want to keep my flat tidy.

2 Do I really want to be disciplined in this area or am I only saying so to please others or get them 'off my back'?
Well, my mother is appalled with the state of my flat. I know she's right.

3 Why do I want to be disciplined in this area?
I don't want my family and friends to think I am a dirty person.

4 Which values underpin my reasons and how important are these

values in my life, on a scale from 0 = no importance to 10 = great importance?
Approval = 7
Tidiness = 1
5 How committed am I to working to develop and maintain self-discipline in this area, on a scale from 0 = no commitment to 10 = full commitment?
Commitment = 3

Sandra's example discussed   Sandra has selected an area of self-discipline that is easier to develop and maintain than Harry's, but the main problem in Sandra's case is that her personal motivation to work towards her stated goal is low. Note the way she has answered Question 2. She says that her mother is appalled at the state of her flat, and the way she says, 'I know she is right,' indicates a grudging acceptance of a problem which in all probability she would not see as a problem if her mother (and others) made no reference to it. Sandra needs to ask herself the following question: 'If my mother and others made no comment on the state of my flat and did not care one way or the other how tidy it was, would I still wish to be more self-disciplined in this area?' My hunch is that Sandra would answer 'no' to this question. If she were to answer 'yes' to it, then she may have to confront the issue of the very low rating she gave to 'tidiness' in response to Question 4.

If we consider the strength of her value ratings we see that having the approval of her family and friends is rated relatively highly ('7'). The real issue, though, is whether such a rating is sufficient to sustain Sandra when the going gets tough in her area of self-discipline. It is important to note in this respect that, as a general rule, you are more likely to achieve and maintain self-discipline in an area where you have intrinsic motivation (i.e. where the reasons for self-discipline are important to you) than when you have extrinsic motivation (i.e. where the reasons for self-discipline are important to others). In this respect, note Sandra's very low rating of tidiness as an intrinsic value ('1'). This predicts self-discipline failure.

Finally, note that Sandra's stated level of commitment to self-discipline in this area is low ('3') and thus she will be unlikely to sustain self-discipline over time. If Sandra is to tidy her flat, she will tend to do this before visits from family or friends rather than generally, and thus she needs to develop what might be called 'situationally based' self-discipline in this area. Thus, Sandra's revised goal might be: 'I want to tidy my flat the night before family and friends come to visit.'

Barbara's example

1   In which area of my life do I want to be more disciplined?
    I want to exercise regularly.
2   Do I really want to be disciplined in this area or am I only saying so
    to please others or get them 'off my back'?
    I want to do this for myself. Nobody else is expressing an opinion.
3   Why do I want to be disciplined in this area?
    I want to establish and maintain a good level of health and fitness.
4   Which values underpin my reasons and how important are these
    values in my life, on a scale from 0 = no importance to 10 = great
    importance?
    Health = 5
    Fitness = 4
    Appearance = 3
5   How committed am I to working to develop and maintain self-dis-
    cipline in this area, on a scale from 0 = no commitment to 10 = full
    commitment?
    Commitment = 9

Barbara's example discussed   Barbara has selected an area of self-
discipline that is fairly difficult to develop and maintain. Consequently,
she needs a relatively high level of commitment and this level needs to
be underpinned by values that will serve to sustain Barbara when the
going gets tough.

It is promising that Barbara's motivation is intrinsic (i.e. she wants
to exercise for herself) rather than extrinsic (i.e. wanting to exercise for
others). However, her biggest problem lies in the discrepancy between
the strength of her ratings of the values that underpin her decision to
exercise regularly (which are moderate or below – '5', '4' and '3') and
her rating of her commitment to work towards achieving and sus-
taining regular exercise (which is high, '9'). In such cases, the person
has overestimated her level of commitment.

If Barbara is truly to develop a high commitment to regular exercise rather than a moderate one, she will have to add to the numbers
of moderately strong values that underpin her decision to strive for
greater self-discipline in this area and/or develop some stronger underpinning values.

Summary suggestions for setting goals for self-discipline

In summary, if you are going to target an area in which to become self-
disciplined, you will increase your chances of success if you:

1   select an area in which you (rather than others) seek change;
2   select an area where your motivation for change is intrinsic rather
    than extrinsic;

3 ensure that strong values underpin the reasons for greater self-discipline;
4 select an area of self-discipline where your level of commitment is high and accurately reflects your strong values.

Am I worth doing it for?

You may conclude that it is worth it to you to work towards developing self-discipline, but still not do so. This may well be the case because you do not think that you yourself are worth developing self-discipline for. In common parlance, you have low self-esteem.

As I have shown in my book *How to Accept Yourself* (Sheldon Press, 1999), low self-esteem (or LSE) comes in many forms. I will discuss three types of LSE here, as they relate to impediments to the development of self-discipline, and suggest how to address this problem.

Worthlessness

If you believe that you are worthless, you will not work to develop self-discipline because you think that you are not worth the effort. If you have children, it is very unlikely that you would teach them such a philosophy. Imagine that your children come home from school and that you discourage them from doing their homework because you tell them they are worthless and don't deserve to get on in life! The chances are that you wouldn't do that, would you? And yet this is precisely how you treat yourself if you are reluctant to develop self-discipline because you think you are not worth doing it for.

Worthlessness is, at bottom, a belief. In thinking that you are worthless, you are assigning a negative global rating to yourself, and in doing so you are ignoring your complexity and humanity. With respect to your complexity, you are far too complex to merit a single global rating that accounts for you as a unique individual. Yes, you may have your faults, but when you say that you are worthless you are focusing on these faults and concluding that you are worthless for having these faults. This is a highly illogical overgeneralization, isn't it? In reality, you have many different aspects to you and, as with all other humans, these are likely to be negative, positive and neutral. You are human, after all, and the essence of being human is that you are fallible. If you accept yourself for being fallible and stop demanding that you must not have faults, then you will begin to accept yourself. In doing so, you will address these faults (like lack of self-discipline), free from the interfering monologue of worthlessness.

If worthlessness is a significant problem for you, you would do well to read and follow the step-by-step exercises that I present in my book *How to Accept Yourself.* However, for the present purposes, my major suggestion is this. Act *as if* you accept yourself! Even though you do not feel it yet, act as if you are worth making the effort for and engage in a sustained programme designed to develop self-discipline. If you do so and periodically remind yourself that you are fallible, not worthless (even though you don't feel it yet), then you will find that after a while you will begin to feel differently about yourself. This won't happen overnight, to be sure, but it will happen if you act and think that you are worth making the effort for. Try it and see.

'I am bad'

When you believe that you are bad, it is usually because you have broken your moral code and have a rigid and extreme view of yourself for breaking that code. You believe that you absolutely should not have done what you did or absolutely should have done what you did not do, and that you are bad through and through for acting badly. As with worthlessness, you do not think that you deserve to develop self-discipline. Indeed, you may engage in self-undisciplined behaviour either because you wish to punish yourself for being bad or to forget how bad you are.

In order to deal with the idea that you are bad, you need to do the following:

1 Accept responsibility for breaking your moral code.
2 Show yourself that while what you did was bad (if indeed it was), this does not prove you are bad as a person. When you think you are bad for breaking your moral code, you are making the part–whole error, where you define the whole of yourself by one of your parts. Instead, show yourself, as before, that you are a fallible human being who is not immune from wrongdoing and that being fallible incorporates this wrongdoing. When you have done this you will be in a better position to look again at what you did (or failed to do) with a greater sense of compassion and understanding, while all the time taking full responsibility for your behaviour.
3 As before, act as if you are not a bad person but a fallible person who can still benefit from self-discipline, and remember that you do not have to punish yourself or engage in self-undisciplined behaviour to blot out your badness. If you consistently do this, it will help you to develop self-acceptance which will, in turn, encourage you to pursue self-discipline.

Selflessness

When you have a selfless philosophy, you believe that you come last and that you can only focus on your desires and priorities when others with whom you are concerned have been helped to satisfy their desires and meet their priorities, particularly by you. The problem with this philosophy is twofold. First, it reflects a low opinion of yourself, one that can only be raised by helping others rather than yourself. Second, since it is unlikely that the desires and priorities of everyone with whom you are concerned will be fully met at any one time, you never really get round to focusing on what is important to you. With respect to your self-discipline goals, this means that you never quite get round to going to the gym, for example, because something always crops up concerning what others want which has greater priority for you.

In order to deal with the philosophy of selflessness, you need to do the following:

1　Realize that when you hold a philosophy of selflessness you think that your worth is derived from making sure that others are looked after. This is a mistake because you will always be focused on others and rarely on yourself, which means effectively that you will not devote sufficient time to your self-discipline goals. In doing so, you will implicitly train others to seek help from you rather than to do things for themselves. Also, you will serve as a poor role model for others. You will teach them that it is wrong to look after themselves and that it is right to look after others, as I will discuss below.

2　You need to see clearly that there is a healthy alternative to selflessness. This is known as the philosophy of self-care. This alternative philosophy spells out that it is healthy to take care of yourself as well as to take care of others. Indeed, it points out that if you are taking care of others first, then the consequence is that they are putting themselves first and you are putting them first. As a result, who is putting you first? That's right – *nobody*! So if you don't look after yourself, it is likely that nobody will. Once you have grasped this point intellectually, the only way that you will internalize it is to put it into practice. So set your self-discipline goals and make it a priority to work towards these goals *before* you tend to others. This will 'feel' strange and all wrong at first. But if you act on the principle of self-care even though it 'feels' all wrong, you will eventually reach the point when it 'feels' right.

3　One of the biggest obstacles to you pursuing your self-discipline goals when you hold a philosophy of selflessness is that you think that putting yourself first means that you are a selfish person. This does not hold up to scrutiny. If you look carefully at what selfishness means, you will see that it tends to mean pursuing your interests compulsively while cynically disregarding the interests of others. This hardly reflects your behaviour, particularly when you tend to the opposite, i.e. compulsively helping others to pursue their interests while cynically disregarding your own! Even if you do act selfishly at times by this definition, does this make you a selfish person? Again, hardly, since if you were a selfish person you would rarely consider the interests of others as you ruthlessly pursued your own agenda in much of your life. And yet this is what people who adhere to a principle of selflessness fear – that if they put themselves first they will turn into a selfish person. Realize that this is hardly likely and that a philosophy of self-care means that while you will basically care for yourself, you will, at times, put others' interests before your own. A philosophy of self-care is at its heart flexible and means that, being human, you may even act selfishly. If so, this does not mean you are a selfish person: it is only evidence of your fallibility and that you have made an error of judgement that you can reflect upon and learn from. While it is important that you understand this, you will only truly believe it if you act on it. So again make a commitment to look after yourself by setting and pursuing your self-discipline goals before helping others to pursue their interests.

If you follow the guidelines that I have put forward in this section then you will be able to answer the question 'Am I worth being self-disciplined for?' with a resounding 'Yes!'

After you have established that your self-discipline goals are worth pursuing and decided that you can pursue them because you are worth doing it for, it is important that you become aware of and carry out an audit of your self-undisciplined behaviour. This is the subject of the next chapter.

4

Become aware of and make an audit of your self-undisciplined behaviour

Become aware of your self-indiscipline

The first step that you need to take if you are to be disciplined is to become aware of your self-indiscipline. This is more difficult than it sounds, for a number of reasons, most of which stem from the workings of your short-term self (STS).

- You may not label your unhealthy behaviour as unhealthy behaviour (e.g. if you smoke, you may not label this as unhealthy).
- You may tend to underestimate the extent of your unhealthy behaviour even if you do label it as such (e.g. if you smoke, you may underestimate the number of cigarettes that you smoke per day).
- You may tend to minimize the effects of your unhealthy behaviour (e.g. if you smoke, you may think that the consequences of smoking are less serious than they actually are).
- If you experience such negative effects, you may fail to attribute these effects to the unhealthy behaviour (e.g. if you smoke and you have successive chest infections, you may wrongly attribute these to a virus that is 'going around').

If you are to give yourself a chance of becoming self-disciplined, you need to deal effectively with your rationalizations and minimizations. To do so, you will have to be honest with yourself. Ask yourself if you are being truthful to yourself or lying to yourself. Here is one way of telling the difference. It is what I call the 'Self-Discipline Parenting Response' technique. Here is how to use this technique with reference to the above example of your smoking behaviour.

Imagine that your adolescent or adult offspring has come to you for help with giving up smoking. Answer the following questions:

- Would you encourage her (in this case) not to regard her smoking behaviour as unhealthy?
- Would you encourage her to underestimate her smoking behaviour?
- Would you encourage her to underestimate the negative effects of smoking?

- Would you encourage her to attribute these effects to a virus rather than to smoking?
- In short, would you discourage her from giving up smoking?

If the answers to these questions are 'no', you know that you are deceiving yourself about the extent of your own indiscipline. Realize that this deception is a major block to becoming fully aware of your self-undisciplined behaviour and that only a decision to be fully honest with yourself will sustain you in the long arduous journey to developing and maintaining self-discipline.

Once you have addressed this block, your long-term self (LTS) can do its work in helping you to become fully aware of the problem.

Develop awareness of your self-undisciplined behaviour and its self-disciplined alternative

Before you embark on developing self-discipline in the chosen area of your life, it is important that you develop awareness of your existing self-undisciplined behaviour and the self-disciplined alternative that you wish to develop. This involves you collecting comprehensive information on the problem and the solution.

Two types of self-indiscipline

When you focus on your self-undisciplined behaviour, you need to be aware of which type of self-indiscipline you are currently showing. There are basically two types of self-indiscipline:

1 the presence of self-undisciplined behaviour
2 the absence of self-disciplined behaviour.

You may think that these two types of self-indiscipline are the same, but they are not.

The presence of self-undisciplined behaviour

Self-indiscipline characterized by the presence of self-undisciplined behaviour occurs, as the name implies, when you act in ways that are self-undisciplined. Here, behaviour is excessive and generally defeats the goals that your LTS has identified. Examples of such behaviour include overeating, smoking, drinking to excess and drug-taking. All these activities are pleasurable (in the short term), but interfere with your long-term healthy functioning and with your striving towards your long-term self-discipline goals.

Another example of the presence of self-undisciplined behaviour that seems different, but isn't, is overwork. Many so-called workaholics work too much and this interferes with their family life. They get a buzz from working and often feel irritable when they are not doing something that in their minds is not productive (i.e. work-related).

Monitoring the presence of self-undisciplined behaviour   In order to monitor your self-undisciplined behaviour, I suggest that you need to use the following scheme.

Date	Time	Situation	Alone/with others	Description of self-undisciplined behaviour

The purpose of this scheme is twofold. First, it helps you to focus your observations. Rooting your observations in specific dates, times and situations helps you to do this. Second, it helps you to see that your self-undisciplined behaviour is linked to contexts both physical and interpersonal, and that it does not happen 'out of the blue'.

Table 4 is an example of self-monitoring of self-undisciplined behaviour by Ellen, whose target problem is overeating.

Table 4 Ellen's example

Date	Time	Situation	Alone/with others	Description of self-undisciplined behaviour
17/3	6.25 p.m.	Kitchen	Alone	Ate six slices of bread
17/3	7.12 p.m.	Kitchen	Alone	Ate five Cream Crackers
17/3	7.30 p.m.	Lounge	With David	Ate one Mars bar watching TV
17/3	8.03 p.m.	Lounge	With David	Ate half a Crunchie bar watching TV

Ellen's example discussed   Ellen's goal is to eat three good meals a day and not to eat between meals. Her monitoring form indicates two patterns. First, when she is alone in her kitchen she eats savoury food, and second, when she is with her partner she eats sweet food. Later, in Chapters 8 and 12, we will return to Ellen's example and I will show how I helped her to understand the factors underlying her self-undisciplined behaviour.

The absence of self-disciplined behaviour   Self-indiscipline characterized by the absence of self-disciplined behaviour occurs, as again the name implies, when you fail to act in ways that are self-disciplined. Here, you fail to act in ways that are necessary to achieve your healthy goals. Failure to keep to an exercise regime would be a typical example of this form of self-indiscipline.

Monitoring the absence of self-disciplined behaviour In order to monitor your self-undisciplined behaviour, you need to be aware of times when you could have acted in a disciplined way but didn't. In doing so, I suggest that you need to use the following scheme.

Date	Time	Planned self-disciplined behaviour	Planned situation	What I actually did	Situation	Alone/with others

The purpose of this scheme is twofold. First, it again helps you to focus your observations. Second, it helps you to see the relationship between your lack of self-disciplined behaviour and the physical and interpersonal contexts that you are in. There are a number of differences between this form and the form that you used to monitor your self-undisciplined behaviour. On the latter, you note your self-undisciplined behaviour whenever and wherever it occurs, but on the form to monitor your absence of self-disciplined behaviour, the 'date' and 'time' sections represent precisely when you had planned to carry out the planned self-disciplined behaviour, which is indicated under its own heading. In addition, the 'planned situation' section indicates where you intended to carry out the planned self-disciplined behaviour. The

Table 5 Colin's example

Date	Time	Planned self-disciplined behaviour	Planned situation	What I actually did	Situation	Alone/with others
4/6	7 p.m.	Working on my essay (three hours)	Study	Tidied my room	Study	Alone
5/6	7 p.m.	Working on my essay (three hours)	Study	Socialized and got drunk	Pub	With mates
6/6	7 p.m.	Working on my essay (three hours)	Study	Listened to iPod and had sex	Study	With Suzy
7/6	7 p.m.	Working on my essay (three hours)	Study	Worked on essay for 30 mins and then got stoned	Study	Alone
8/6	7 p.m.	Working on my essay (three hours)	Study	Listened to CDs and got stoned	Study	Alone

other sections reflect what you actually did, and where you were and who you were with when you did it.

Table 5 is an example of self-monitoring of self-undisciplined behaviour by Colin, whose planned self-disciplined behaviour is working on his essay.

Colin's example discussed   In looking at Colin's form in Table 5, it becomes clear that there is no simple pattern to explain his procrastination on working on his essay (his target self-disciplined behaviour). He puts off doing his work when he is alone and when he is with other people, when he is in his study and when he is not. We will have to look more deeply into the factors that come into play which lead Colin to procrastinate, and we will do this in Chapter 5.

Serious self-indiscipline

Serious self-indiscipline occurs when you display both the presence of self-undisciplined behaviour and the absence of self-disciplined behaviour in an area that poses a serious threat to your physical and/ or psychological health, as in Malcolm's example. In monitoring such serious self-discipline, you need to use both forms – one for the presence of self-disciplined behaviour and the other for the absence of self-disciplined behaviour.

Malcolm's example

At his annual health check, it was discovered that Malcolm's blood pressure and cholesterol levels were seriously elevated and posed a serious risk to his physical health. In no uncertain terms, Malcolm's physician told him that if he did not modify his eating and drinking habits and exercise regularly, then he was a good candidate for a heart attack in the not too distant future. Malcolm's response to this news was to ignore the warning, and he continued with his high cholesterol diet and 12 pints of beer a day routine (the presence of self-undisciplined behaviour) and categorically refused to do any exercise (the absence of self-disciplined behaviour).

If you demonstrate serious self-indiscipline, you need more help than I can provide you in a book of this nature. You need professional help, and it is worth discussing this with your doctor in the first instance.

Carry out a thorough audit of your self-undisciplined behaviour and its self-disciplined alternative

Before you embark on developing self-discipline in the chosen area of your life, it is important that you carry out a thorough audit of your existing self-undisciplined behaviour and the self-disciplined alternative that you wish to develop. Conducting a thorough audit of your self-undisciplined behaviour and its disciplined alternative involves you looking at the costs and benefits of the alternatives available to you, and others involved, from short-term and long-term perspectives.

The purpose of an audit and its four major elements

The purpose of conducting an audit of your current self-indiscipline and your desired state of self-discipline is twofold. First, it helps you to identify factors that encourage you to develop self-discipline and those that serve as obstacles to you developing it in your selected area.

There are four elements to such an audit:

- the costs of self-undisciplined behaviour
- the perceived advantages of self-undisciplined behaviour
- the advantages of self-disciplined behaviour
- the perceived costs of self-disciplined behaviour.

As I said earlier, when you carry out an audit you consider each of the above from a short-term perspective and a long-term perspective, from the standpoint of yourself and that of significant others involved.

I will discuss how you use such information later in the book.

Develop a list of the costs of self-undisciplined behaviour

A major part of an audit on self-indiscipline is the development of a comprehensive list of the costs of the self-undisciplined behaviour that you have targeted for change.

There are four elements to a cost audit of self-undisciplined behaviour:

- short-term costs to yourself
- long-term costs to yourself
- short-term costs to others involved
- long-term costs to others involved.

What follows is a cost audit that Glenda did on her target self-undisciplined behaviour: smoking.

Audit of the costs of smoking: Glenda's example
Short-term costs to myself
- I smell like an ashtray.
- I drink more when I smoke.
- My throat feels sore straight after smoking.
- Because I can only smoke outside, I am more vulnerable to colds and flu in the winter.

Long-term costs to myself
- I am making myself more vulnerable to a whole host of diseases.

- I am spending far too much money on cigarettes, money that I could spend more productively or even save or invest.
- I am losing my sense of taste.
- I am unfit and breathless and don't feel like exercising when I smoke.

Short-term costs to others involved
- My children get very upset when they see or know that I have been smoking.
- I upset people who object to others smoking.

Long-term costs to others involved
- My children will be deprived of their mother if I get ill or die prematurely from smoking-related diseases.
- My children will be worried in the long term about me.
- I may well be harming my children with passive smoke when I smoke outdoors but in their presence.

Develop a list of the perceived advantages of self-undisciplined behaviour

Part of a comprehensive audit of self-indiscipline involves you identifying what you (or more accurately your short-term self) see as the advantages of your self-undisciplined behaviour. These advantages represent your STS's preoccupation with short-term pleasure.

There are four elements to an audit of the perceived advantages of self-undisciplined behaviour:

- short-term advantages to yourself
- long-term advantages to yourself
- short-term advantages to others involved
- long-term advantages to others involved.

Later I will show you how your LTS can respond to these perceived advantages, charged as it is with your long-term well-being.

This is Glenda's audit of the perceived advantages of smoking.

Audit of the perceived advantages of smoking: Glenda's example
Short-term advantages to myself
- It makes me feel and look cool.
- I feel part of the group when I am with my friends who smoke.

Long-term advantages to myself
- As a smoker I think of myself as bohemian.

Short-term advantages to others involved
- When I smoke with my smoking friends they feel more comfortable.

Long-term advantages to others involved
- My smoking friends will not feel that I have betrayed them if I keep smoking.

Develop a list of the advantages of self-disciplined behaviour

When a person's goal is to stop engaging in self-undisciplined behaviour like smoking, it is the absence of self-undisciplined behaviour that is the goal. It is easier to strive towards the presence of a desired state than towards the absence of an undesired state, and therefore whenever possible it is helpful to set as a goal the presence of self-disciplined behaviour rather than the absence of self-undisciplined behaviour. However, for some people this just does not make sense and in the case of Glenda, as we can see below, the desired state was 'not smoking'.

Audit of the perceived advantages of not smoking: Glenda's example
Short-term advantages to myself
- I smell nicer when I don't smoke.
- I like the feeling of being in control when I don't smoke.
- I feel proud when my kids are proud of me when I don't smoke.

Long-term advantages to myself
- Increased fitness.
- Better health.
- Saves money.
- Sets a good example for my kids.

Short-term advantages to others involved
- My kids feel proud when I don't smoke.
- Most people are happier being around me when I don't smoke.

Long-term advantages to others involved
- I will live longer and therefore will not deprive my children of their mother.
- My children will not be worried about me in the long term if I give up smoking.
- My children will be healthier when I give up smoking since they will not have to be exposed to any passive smoking.
- My kids can see that it is possible to give up bad habits.

Develop a list of the perceived costs of self-disciplined behaviour

The final audit that you need to take involves you identifying the costs that you think are involved with respect to your self-disciplined behaviour. Again, this list emanates from your STS.

There are four elements to an audit of the perceived costs of disciplined behaviour:

- short-term costs to yourself
- long-term costs to yourself
- short-term costs to others involved
- long-term costs to others involved.

What follows is an audit of the perceived costs involved with not smoking.

Audit of the perceived costs of not smoking: Glenda's example
Short-term costs to myself
- I feel edgy when I don't smoke.
- I get more colds when I don't smoke.
- My smoking buddies treat me as a bit of an outcast.

Long-term costs to myself
- I would see myself as more staid, less bohemian, if I were to give up smoking.

Short-term costs to others involved
- I make my smoking buddies uncomfortable if, when I am with them, I don't smoke and they do.

Long-term costs to others involved
- My smoking buddies will feel betrayed if I stop smoking.

Respond to the perceived advantages of self-undisciplined behaviour and the perceived costs of self-disciplined behaviour

Once you have conducted a thorough audit of your self-undisciplined behaviour and your desired self-disciplined alternative, you need to use your LTS to help you to respond to what you see as the advantages of your current self-undisciplined behaviour and the disadvantages of your desired self-disciplined behaviour. Let me consider these one at a time.

Respond to the perceived advantages of self-undisciplined behaviour

When you decide to target your self-undisciplined behaviour for change it is because you have sensed that it is not working for you. When you conduct an audit and focus on the disadvantages of this self-undisciplined behaviour and the advantages of the self-disciplined alternative, you unpack this sense and provide yourself with reasons to help you in your quest towards self-discipline.

When you outline what you see as the advantages of your self-undisciplined behaviour, you are identifying a set of the obstacles that need to be addressed if you are to develop self-discipline. One way of doing this is to respond to these obstacles. When you do so, it is useful to do one or more of the following:

- Respond to any errors of fact or logic.

- Point out how you can achieve the advantages of your current self-undisciplined behaviour in ways that are healthier for you.
- Remind yourself that engaging in the advantages of your self-undisciplined behaviour is not worth it to you.

Here is how Glenda responded to the advantages that she identified with respect to smoking, using some of the arguments listed above.

Perceived advantages of smoking and response: Glenda's example
Short-term advantages to myself

- It makes me feel and look cool.
  Response: That may be the case, but I look pretty good without smoking. And if smoking does make me look cool, looking cool isn't worth dying for!

- I feel part of the group when I am with my friends who smoke.
  Response: But I can feel a part of this group without smoking. It's the conversation that is important here and not the smoking. But even if the smoking is the important ingredient here, once again it's not worth dying for.

Long-term advantages to myself

- As a smoker I think of myself as bohemian.
  Response: But I can still be bohemian in other ways if I want to and not smoke. I can dress in a bohemian style. There are no government health warnings on clothing.

Short-term advantages to others involved

- When I smoke with my smoking friends they feel more comfortable.
  Response: If this is true, then I am not prepared to jeopardize my health to make them feel momentarily comfortable. They can still be friends with me even if I don't smoke.

Long-term advantages to others involved

- My smoking friends will not feel that I have betrayed them if I keep smoking.
  Response: If this is true, then a friendship based on me smoking is not for me.

Respond to the perceived disadvantages of self-disciplined behaviour

When you outline what you see as the disadvantages of your desired self-disciplined behaviour, you are identifying another set of obstacles that need to be addressed if you are to develop self-discipline. Again, responding to these obstacles using the following arguments is one way of dealing with them.

- Respond to any errors of fact or logic.

- Point out how you can avoid the disadvantages of your desired self-disciplined behaviour in ways that are healthier for you.
- Remind yourself that engaging in the disadvantages of your desired self-disciplined behaviour is not worth it to you.

Here is how Glenda responded to the disadvantages that she identified with respect to not smoking, using some of the arguments listed above.

Perceived costs of not smoking and response: Glenda's example
Short-term costs to myself
- I feel edgy when I don't smoke.
  Response: There is no getting away with this, but if I tolerate this edginess it will gradually go.

- I get more colds when I don't smoke.
  Response: This is my system's way of adjusting to being without nicotine. It won't last.

- My smoking buddies treat me as a bit of an outcast.
  Response: If this is true, I will discuss it with them. If they ostracize me it is a price worth paying.

Long-term costs to myself
- I would see myself as more staid, less bohemian, if I were to give up smoking.
  Response: I can be bohemian in other ways, if that is important to me. I don't have to link this aspect of myself with smoking.

Short-term costs to others involved
- I make my smoking buddies uncomfortable if, when I am with them, I don't smoke and they do.
  Response: I am not sure that this is true so I need to check it out with them. However, if it is true, then that is a small price to pay for giving up smoking.

Long-term costs to others involved
- My smoking buddies will feel betrayed if I stop smoking.
  Response: Again, I will need to check this out with them. If it is true then they are reacting as if we have made a formal pact that nobody will ever leave the 'smoking' club. That is ridiculous. This is how they may feel, but if it is I really don't want to be friends with people who make friendship dependent on a life-threatening habit.

In Appendices 2–5, you will find blanks of the forms that you need to complete in developing awareness of and conducting an audit of your self-undisciplined behaviour and your self-disciplined alternative, and in responding to the perceived advantages of self-undisciplined behaviour and the perceived costs of self-disciplined behaviour.

Part 3

When self-discipline involves taking action

In this book, I will deal with two types of self-discipline: self-discipline which involves taking disciplined action, and self-discipline which involves refraining from taking self-undisciplined action. While there are features both types have in common, I will deal with them one at a time because they differ in important respects. In this part of the book, I will deal with self-discipline which involves taking disciplined action, and discuss the important issues that you need to consider when working towards developing this type of self-discipline. In doing so, I will illustrate my points, where relevant, with reference to the example of Colin, whose self-disciplined behavioural target was working on his essay. In the following part of the book, I will discuss self-discipline which involves refraining from taking self-undisciplined action.

5

Plan and prepare for self-disciplined action

If your target is to develop self-discipline which involves taking disciplined action, you need to make effective plans and properly prepare yourself in order to maximize the chances that you will develop this type of self-discipline. If you rely on your ability in the moment to act in a self-disciplined manner without proper planning and preparation, you will then increase the chances that you will act in a self-undisciplined way.

The following are important elements to effective planning and preparation.

Consider the components of the task and focus on one component at a time

There may be some self-disciplined tasks that are fairly simple and do not need breaking down into their component parts. Having an early night is one task that is fairly simple, as is running, although both these tasks have associated activities that have to be completed first (e.g. having an early night involves removing one's day clothes, getting into one's night apparel, washing and cleaning one's teeth; running involves dressing in the right clothes, doing warm-up exercises).

However, other self-disciplined tasks are more complex and do need breaking down into their component parts (known as sub-tasks). For example, let's suppose that writing a short story is your self-disciplined task. Before you actually put pen to paper, you will need to do some or all of the following sub-tasks:

- Brainstorm the content of your storyline.
- Work on the details of the storyline.
- Do appropriate research.
- Choose your characters carefully.
- Flesh out your characters.
- Develop a writing plan.
- Do a first draft.
- Do subsequent drafts.
- Get feedback from others, if appropriate.

- Write final draft.

When you are planning to write a short story, then, you need to consider the components of the main task and then focus on one sub-task at a time. When a mountain climber plans to climb a mountain, she looks at the mountain, divides up the climb and then focuses on one 'sub-climb' at a time. The same applies to writing a short story. Divide up the task and then focus on one sub-task at a time.

Undertake a skills audit and take remedial action if necessary

As part of your planning and preparation, you need to consider your targeted self-disciplined task and its component parts and evaluate which skills they involve. Then you need to consider whether or not you have these skills in your skill repertoire. If you don't have a particular skill that you need to complete the task or, more commonly, one of the sub-tasks, then you need to acquire this skill before embarking on the task (or relevant sub-task).

You need to be careful here since there are two traps. First, you may use this as an excuse to put off doing the task. Here, you actually have the skill in your skill repertoire, but you persuade yourself that you don't. Second, you may think that you need to be more competent at the task than you are before starting it. I consider this below. As elsewhere, you need to be honest with yourself and recognize that you are deceiving yourself in the first instance and being overly demanding in the second.

Allocate time to a task

I once counselled a man who had sought my help for his anger problem. One of the contributing factors to his anger was his refusal to allocate more time to a task than he believed it should ideally take. For example, he worked in the City, and ideally it should have taken him 20 minutes to reach Waterloo station from his office at the end of a working day, to catch his train home to suburbia. In fact, he was only able to do this if everything was in his favour. As you can imagine, with evening rush-hour in London, things rarely were ideal and he routinely faced delays to his journey. These delays meant that he frequently missed his train, and this made him furious. He would complain long and hard about London Underground's failings, and the unreasonable behaviour of commuters who would not walk on the 'correct' side of the road and who took their time in getting on and off tube trains. One thing that he categorically refused to do was to devote more time to his journey ... with predictable results!

The reason that I have quoted this example is to show you two things. First, it is very important to consider the task that you are focusing on and then come to a judgement concerning how much time it will take you to carry out this task. Second, and perhaps more importantly, as the example with my client above shows it is very important to allocate more time than you think the task will actually take to cover unforeseen eventualities.

There are three areas where you need to consider allocating time to tasks.

1 Allocate time to the task as a whole. Here you need to take into account any relevant external deadlines.
2 Allocate time to each of the relevant sub-tasks.
3 Allocate time to that aspect of the task that you are going to do 'in one sitting', by which I mean a single block of time you have chosen to carry out self-disciplined activity (e.g. write a briefing report from 10 a.m. to 12 noon on a Friday morning).

I will illustrate these points when discussing Colin's example – see below.

Choose a favourable time

When you plan to act in a self-disciplined manner, you will increase the chances of doing so if you choose a favourable time to carry out such behaviour. If you choose a time that is inconvenient for you, then you may well find it harder to act in a self-disciplined manner. For example, let's suppose that you have targeted exercise as your self-discipline goal. You will increase your chances of carrying out such exercise if you choose a time to do so when there are no competing activities to distract you. Thus, I exercise first thing in the morning, when I have little else to do. If I were to plan to exercise later in the day, then I might well find it harder to do because there would be other calls on my time (e.g. emails to answer, telephone calls to take, and other tasks to do).

Choose a favourable setting

You can increase the chances that you will act in a self-disciplined manner if you choose a setting which is likely to facilitate this behaviour rather than inhibit it. What constitutes a favourable setting will vary from person to person. People tend to vary according to what are favourable settings for them in this respect. Let me take writing as an example. Some people prefer to write in a quiet setting, free from any distractions. Others prefer to write in an environment where there is some background noise. Thus, I like writing in coffee bars where there is sufficient background noise to enable me to concentrate on the task at hand. I actually find it very difficult to concentrate on writing in a very quiet environment. Extrapolating from my personal example, I suggest that you focus on the task that you have to perform, and consider the environment in which you are most likely to perform it.

Have relevant resources available

When you are planning to carry out a self-disciplined task, it is important that you have to hand those resources that you need in order to perform the task. It is important that you do this *before* you begin the task at the agreed time. Otherwise, you may be tempted to spend time gathering these resources, thinking that you are doing the task while, in reality, you are avoiding it. I call this 'pseudo work'. For example, let us revisit the episode where Colin tidied his study instead of writing his essay. If doing this helped enable Colin to gather the resources that he needed to work on his essay, then he would do this as part of his preparations and not as part of the task itself. When I plan to do a spell of writing, I make sure that my laptop has enough battery life, that I have the books that I need and, if I need to access the internet, I ensure that I have the relevant website addresses. I do all of these things *before* I start working.

Minimize potential obstacles

I have stressed that an important part of making preparations for self-disciplined action is for you to choose a time and a place which maximize the chances of you actually doing so. It is also important for you to choose a time and a place where potential obstacles to acting in a self-disciplined way are minimized. For example, I mentioned above that I prefer to do my writing in an environment where there is some background noise. Thus, I will often choose a coffee bar in which to write. However, I will not choose to work in a coffee bar where there is a good chance that I may be interrupted by people I know.

I recognize that you cannot always identify obstacles to self-disciplined action in advance. However, with a little bit of foresight, it is possible to anticipate certain events which may serve to prevent you from carrying out your self-disciplined task.

Use imagery rehearsal

Once you have made adequate preparations to carry out your self-disciplined task, you may find it useful to rehearse executing this task in your mind's eye before you do so in reality. The use of such imagery rehearsal is based on the principle that you are more likely to do something once you have pictured yourself doing it in your mind's eye. I suggest two ways of implementing this principle.

Behaviourally based imagery rehearsal

This technique involves you picturing yourself acting in the desired self-disciplined way. I call this technique 'behaviourally based imagery rehearsal' because when you employ it you are just focusing on your behaviour. In doing so, I suggest that you focus particularly on any parts of the process where you experience particular difficulty acting in the desired self-disciplined manner.

Let me illustrate by showing you how Colin used behaviourally based imagery rehearsal. Note, in particular, how Colin used imagery to focus specifically on starting to write his essay.

First, Colin pictured himself the night before, gathering all the materials that he needed to work on the essay. Then, he saw himself rising at 7 a.m., having breakfast, placing a 'please do not disturb' sign on his door, turning off his mobile phone and then sitting down at his desk in his study at 7.30 a.m., ready to work. Next, Colin clearly saw himself picking up his pen and writing the title of the essay and the introduction. He particularly focused on these specific activities because his main problem in implementing his self-discipline strategy was actually starting it. After he saw himself start writing, Colin spent some time picturing himself continuing to write and implementing two short planned coffee breaks of ten minutes each. After each break, Colin imagined himself picking up his pen and continuing to write the essay. Again, notice how Colin focused intently on points in the process where he experienced most difficulty.

Cognitive behavioural imagery rehearsal

This second technique involves you picturing yourself both acting in the desired self-disciplined way and thinking various things that are designed to aid your implementation of this behaviour. I call this 'cognitive behavioural imagery rehearsal' because when you employ it you are focusing on your behaviour and your thinking. Again, as you do so I suggest that you especially focus on any parts of the process where you experience particular difficulty acting in the desired self-disciplined manner.

There are two types of thinking that are especially useful in the imagery rehearsal process. They are self-instructions and belief-challenging thoughts.

Self-instructions Self-instructions are verbal instructions you give yourself to act in a certain way. For example, Colin told himself to put a 'please do not disturb' sign on the door before he did so. This is a self-instruction. Colin then imagined himself putting the sign up. While, in this context, self-instructions are prompts to action in imagery, they can also be used as prompts to action in real life.

'Healthy belief' rehearsal   As the name implies, 'healthy belief' rehearsal is thinking that is designed to practise healthy beliefs at points where the presence of unhealthy beliefs would normally interfere with your self-disciplined behaviour. For example, in his use of cognitive–behavioural imagery rehearsal Colin used 'healthy belief' rehearsal (i.e. 'Starting is uncomfortable but it is in my interests to do so') to help him start his essay (in his imagination) when the existence of an unhealthy belief (i.e. 'I have to be comfortable before I start writing my essay') would normally have prevented him from so doing.

Helping Colin to prepare and plan to take action

Let me now illustrate these points by discussing how I helped Colin to make relevant plans and preparations to work on his essay, on which he had previously procrastinated.

Consider the components of the task and focus on one component at a time

I helped Colin to focus on his essay and all the things that he needed to do to end up with a good piece of work. Together we came up with the following list:

- Make an essay plan.
- Gather the books and articles needed.
- Use the plan to guide my reading.
- Read the material.
- Adjust the essay plan on the basis of my reading.
- Write the first draft.
- Read and edit first draft.
- Write the final draft.

I helped Colin to see that the task of writing his essay depended on him doing a number of prior sub-tasks which influenced its success. I then helped Colin to focus on and do one sub-task at a time. In discussing his approach, I will focus on the first draft of his essay.

Undertake a skills audit and take remedial action if necessary

Colin undertook a thorough audit of his essay-writing skills and concluded that while his note-taking could be better, he had all the necessary skills in his repertoire.

Allocate time to a task

I mentioned earlier in this chapter that you need to think about three ways of allocating time to a task. Here is how Colin addressed this issue. Remember that I suggested that you should allocate more time to a task than you think it will take, given that life isn't perfect and will throw up obstacles that may disrupt your timetable. In doing so, it is important that you don't think of using this extra time as time to do the task. It is there, don't forget, to use only if you need it. If you don't use it, see it as a reward to use for enjoyment! In what follows, notice how Colin made use of this principle of allocating extra time to tasks.

Time allocated to the task as a whole

'The essay I have to write is due in three weeks. I will allocate two and a half weeks to do it and allow an extra half-week in case any unforeseen events occur.'

Time allocated to each sub-task, if relevant

- Make an essay plan = 45 minutes (allow 75 minutes).
- Gather the books and articles needed = two hours (allow three hours).
- Use the plan to guide my reading = ongoing.
- Read the material = five days at four hours per day (allow six days).
- Adjust the essay plan on the basis of my reading = ongoing.
- Write the first draft = three days at four hours per day (allow four days).
- Read and edit first draft = three hours (allow four hours).
- Write the final draft = one day at four hours per day (allow five hours).

Time allocated to task performance in a given sitting

'I will allocate two hours to every "work sitting" and I will allow an extra 30 minutes in case anything untoward happens.'

Choose a favourable time

In discussions with Colin on how he spent his time, it became clear that he liked to spend his evenings with his friends and resented giving up this time to work on his essay. Consequently, he decided that he would get up at 7 a.m. and work on his essay for two hours every morning (from 7.30 a.m. till 9.30 a.m.) after eating his breakfast.

Choose a favourable setting

Colin lived in student accommodation which comprised a small study area and a bedroom. He shared kitchen, bathroom and toilet facilities with other students. Given this, Colin nominated his study area as the best place for him to work on his essay. It was compact and at that time in the morning it was quiet. Colin also had his small hi-fi in the study area, and listening to classical music helped him to concentrate on the essay.

Make available relevant resources

I mentioned above that Colin had used tidying his study as an avoidance manoeuvre. I therefore helped him see the difference between work (i.e. direct work on his essay) and pseudo work (i.e. tidying his study). Since he had to have some writing and reading materials to hand, Colin agreed to have these resources ready the night before, when he went to bed, so he could use them in his designated work period.

Minimize potential obstacles

Although Colin had nominated a time to work on his essay when other students were unlikely to be around, he decided to put a 'do not disturb' sign on his door to discourage visitors who might tempt him away from his work. In addition, he decided to keep his mobile phone switched off while studying, to prevent him from receiving and making calls that would have taken him away from working on his essay.

Use imagery rehearsal

Let me illustrate all these principles by showing you how Colin used imagery rehearsal. First, Colin pictured himself the night before, telling himself, 'OK, get your writing stuff together; books, pens and ruler.' Then he pictured himself getting these materials and placing them next to the space he used for writing. Then he pictured himself doing the following:

- At 7 a.m. he told himself to get up, followed by the action.
- At 7.15 a.m. he saw himself having breakfast.
- Just before 7.30 a.m., he told himself to place the 'please do not disturb' sign on his door and to turn his phone off. He then saw himself performing these actions.
- At 7.30 a.m., Colin told himself to sit down at his desk in his study and begin to work. Then he saw himself actually doing this.

Next, Colin told himself that although starting was difficult it was in his interests to do so, and that once he had started then continuing to write was easier. He then saw himself implementing this by picking up his pen and writing the title of the essay and the introduction. Remember that Colin particularly focused on these activities because his main problem in implementing his self-discipline strategy was starting it.

After he saw himself start writing, Colin spent some time seeing himself continuing to write and implementing two short planned coffee breaks of ten minutes each. After each break, Colin told himself that he could tolerate the discomfort of starting again and then pictured himself picking up the pen and continuing to write his essay. Again, notice how Colin focused intently on points in the process where he experienced most difficulty.

In the next chapter, I will discuss the conditions that you think must exist before you take self-disciplined action and show you how to deal productively with these potential obstacles to self-discipline.

6

Deal with potential obstacles to self-disciplined behaviour

One of the reasons people find it difficult to develop and maintain a self-disciplined approach is that they believe certain conditions have to exist before engaging with a self-disciplined task. This, of course, emanates from the short-term self (STS). In this chapter, I will discuss the most common of these conditions and show you what you need to do to prevent these from becoming obstacles to self-disciplined behaviour.

Motivation

'I have to be motivated to do a task before I do it'

One of the most common conditions that people insist upon before they initiate self-disciplined behaviour is motivation. By motivation, I mean an internal state where the person actively wants to engage in or feels an urge to engage in the self-disciplined activity under consideration.

The main problem with the attitude: 'I have to be motivated to do a task before I do it' is that it is rigid.

The demand for motivation before you act is rigid

When you believe that you have to feel motivated in order to behave in a self-disciplined way, you give yourself no room in which to manoeuvre. Either you are motivated to do the task or you don't do it. As a result, this belief precludes the possibility of you doing the task without motivation. There is nothing wrong at all with wanting to feel motivated before engaging in self-disciplined behaviour, but to demand it means that you are turning a flexible attitude into a rigid one, with only one result ... you will not begin the task until the demanded state of motivation is experienced.

How to deal with your demand for pre-action motivation

The healthy alternative to the rigid belief: 'I have to be motivated to do a task before I do it' is a flexible belief. A flexible belief states what you desire, but acknowledges that you don't have to get what you desire. Here is the flexible belief alternative to the above rigid belief: 'I would like to be motivated to do a task before I do it, but it is not necessary for me to have such motivation. I can begin the task whether I am motivated to do it or not.'

Step 1: Understand why your demand for pre-action motivation is irrational

An irrational idea is one that is false, illogical and unconstructive. Thus, when you find yourself holding a rigid demand for pre-action motivation you need to see the following:

- *It is false*: it is not true that you have to be motivated before you begin to act in a self-disciplined manner. You can start the task without being motivated to start it. Therefore your demand for pre-action motivation is false.

- *It is illogical*: the demand for pre-action motivation is based on the desire for this condition. The full version of your demand is as follows: 'I would like to be motivated before I start the task and therefore I have to be motivated before I start it.' If we break down this full belief into its two parts we can see that the first part: 'I would like to be motivated before I start the task ...' is not rigid, whereas the second part: '... and therefore I have to be motivated before I start it' is rigid. In logic one cannot derive something rigid from something that is not rigid, therefore the demand for pre-action motivation is illogical.

- *It is unconstructive*: when you believe that you have to be motivated to do a task before you do it, you do not engage in the task if you are not motivated to do it. Therefore your demand for pre-action motivation is unconstructive since it prevents you from engaging in behaviour that leads you closer towards your goal. In a phrase, your demand for pre-action motivation is an obstacle to the development of self-discipline.

Step 2: Understand why your flexible desire for pre-action motivation is rational

A rational idea is one that is true, logical and constructive. Thus, you need to see that the flexible alternative to your demand for pre-action motivation – 'I would like to be motivated to do a task before I do it, but it is not necessary for me to have such motivation. I can begin the task whether I am motivated to do it or not' – has these three characteristics.

- *It is true*: it is true that you would like to be motivated before you begin to act in a self-disciplined manner, and it is also true that it is not necessary for you to have such motivation before starting the task. Therefore your flexible desire for pre-action motivation is true.

- *It is logical*: your flexible desire for pre-action motivation has two parts:
  - *Part 1*: 'I would like to be motivated to do a task before I do it ...'
  - *Part 2*: '... but it is not necessary for me to have such motivation. I can begin the task whether I am motivated to do it or not.'

  As you can see, neither of these two parts is rigid and therefore the second non-rigid part logically follows from the first non-rigid part. As such, your flexible preference is logical.

- *It is unconstructive*: when you believe that you would like to be motivated to do a task before you do it, but recognize that it is not necessary for you to have such motivation, you can begin the task whether you are motivated to do it or not. Therefore, your flexible desire for pre-action motivation is constructive since it does not prevent you from engaging in behaviour that leads you closer towards your goal. Indeed, this belief focuses you on taking self-disciplined action whether you feel motivated to take it or not.

Two other problems with the demand for pre-action motivation

There are two other problems with the demand for pre-action motivation:

1 It stops you from learning that you can develop motivation once you have begun the task.
2 It ignores the fact that much self-disciplined behaviour involves discomfort.

The demand for pre-action motivation stops you from learning that you can develop motivation once you have begun the task.

Another problem with the rigid demand for pre-action motivation is that if you allow yourself to be guided by it then you do not learn one important point. This is that if you begin a task without feeling motivated and engage with that task, then some of the time you will begin to experience motivation for and involvement with the task once you are doing it. Of course, this will not always happen, but it does happen enough of the time for you to reformulate your belief. If we incorporate this into your flexible belief concerning pre-action motivation, then we have:

I would like to be motivated to do a task before I do it, but it is not necessary for me to have such motivation. I can begin the task whether I am motivated to do it or not and some of the time I will become motivated and involved in the task once I am doing it.

The demand for pre-action motivation ignores the fact that much self-disciplined behaviour involves discomfort

When you hold a rigid demand for pre-action motivation, you ignore the grim reality that much self-disciplined behaviour involves discomfort. To demand that you feel motivated to engage in uncomfortable tasks is unrealistic. One solution to this problem is to change the focus of your motivation from the task to the outcome of the task. For example, applying this point Colin would concentrate on the fact that he is motivated to have his essay done, rather than motivated to do the task that is necessary to get the essay done.

I frequently encourage my clients to do what they don't want to do in order to achieve what they do want to have done. This is, of course, a variant of encouraging people to put up with short-term pains for long-term gains. So if this is a problem for you, just focus on what you want done and accept the reality that you have to do what you don't want to do in order to achieve your goal.

Anxiety or pressure

'I can't do the task unless I'm anxious or under pressure'

People who believe that they have to feel anxious or be under pressure in order to initiate self-disciplined behaviour are usually operating according to a self-fulfilling prophecy. What normally happens here is as follows. You originally leave a self-disciplined task to the last minute. You then feel anxious or under pressure, and since the idea of not doing the task is more anxiety-provoking than doing it, you do the task, often working long and hard to finish it. If you do finish it, you then strengthen the idea that you can leave things till the last minute and your anxiety or sense of pressure will once again pull you through.

If you operate under this system for a while, you come to believe, quite wrongly as it happens, that you can *only* engage in self-disciplined task activity when you are anxious or under pressure. Indeed, if you try and work when you have plenty of time to do the task, then you won't do it because you have convinced yourself that you need your anxiety (or sense of pressure) to mobilize you.

The demand for pre-action anxiety (or pressure) is rigid

As you have seen in my discussion of the demand for pre-action motivation and as you will repeatedly see when I discuss the other conditions that people insist are in place before they take self-disciplined action, the problems with these demands lie in their rigidity and, in particular, in the effects that such rigidity brings about.

How to deal with your demand for pre-action anxiety

As I explained in the above section on the demand for pre-action motivation, there are two steps in dealing with your demand for pre-action anxiety: showing yourself that this demand is irrational (i.e. unconstructive, illogical and false) and showing yourself that your flexible desire for pre-action anxiety is rational (i.e. constructive, logical and true).

In particular, if you believe that you have to be anxious or under pressure before you engage with the self-disciplined task, then you need to realize that you will not engage with that task until you experience anxiety or a sense of pressure. In believing this, you have to generate anxiety or pressure and you tend to do this by waiting until there is a real chance that you will not complete the task and that you will suffer as a result of your failure to complete it.

You also need to see that this rigid belief rules out the possibility of you working in a more relaxed way. If you try to do this when believing that you must have anxiety to mobilize you, your lack of anxiety will lead you to move away from engaging in the self-disciplined task, supported no doubt by one or more rationalizations which you see as good reasons why you can't get down to work now.

Your rigid demand for pre-action anxiety may also lead you to think that you work best under pressure. To test the validity of this hypothesis, you would need to conduct a controlled experiment comparing your performance and its outcome on two equivalent self-disciplined tasks with the same deadline. First, you would carry out a self-disciplined task while you are anxious, having left the task till the last minute. Then, you would need to carry out the equivalent task starting early and *working diligently* on the task until you have finished it at or before the deadline. My guess would be that you do more efficient and effective work when you start early and work diligently.

When you say that you work best under pressure, you make this conclusion having conducted a very biased experiment. Thus, you observe that you can work quite well under pressure and you also observe that you don't work well when you are not under pressure. Your conclusion that you work best under pressure only shows the impact of your rigid demand for pre-action anxiety. This demand mobilizes you only when you approach a deadline and does not mobilize you when the deadline is far away.

In order to learn just how well you can work a long way in advance of a deadline, you need to do the following:

- You need to agree with yourself a schedule that will enable you to work steadily and finish well ahead of the deadline.
- You need to recognize that you will not 'feel' mobilized to start the task, but if you see such mobilization as a desirable rather than

a mandatory condition, then you will start the task without this 'feeling'.

- Once you have started, throw yourself into the task with as much enthusiasm as you can muster. If you can't feel any enthusiasm, act as if you have it. Remember, you are re-educating yourself to work in a self-disciplined manner without the aid of feelings of anxiety or of being under pressure.

- Continue in this vein until you have finished the task. Remind yourself, when appropriate, of two points. First, you don't need to be anxious or under pressure to engage in a self-disciplined task. Second, it will feel strange working on something when you have plenty of time to do the task, but you can tolerate these strange feelings and work while feeling strange. You will slowly become familiar with the new way of working if you persist with it.

Your flexible preference for pre-action anxiety or pressure before you begin a self-disciplined task is fine and won't get you into trouble as long as you don't act on it. Indeed, even your desire for pre-action anxiety is based on your habit (i.e. 'I work when under pressure, I don't work without it'). Once you have broken the connection between anxiety and work and established a new connection between a more relaxed attitude and work, your desire for pre-action anxiety will change, particularly as you come to appreciate the benefits of the new connection.

Confidence

'I need to feel confident before I do the task'

To some extent we live in a culture that prizes confidence and has little time for lack of confidence. As a result we tend to develop unrealistic expectations about how we are supposed to feel when we engage with a self-disciplined task. When you set a goal in the area of self-discipline, it is usually the case that you have been acting in a self-undisciplined way for quite a while. In pursuing your goal you are asking yourself to act in a self-disciplined manner to which you may be unaccustomed. When you are unaccustomed to doing something, it is realistic to expect yourself to feel *un*confident when you first do it.

The demand for pre-action confidence is rigid, and how to deal with it

If you demand that you have to feel confident doing a task before you do it, then quite simply you will not do it. Why? Because in insisting on pre-action confidence, you will respond to the normal experience of unconfidence under these circumstances with lack of action or avoidance. If you do this, you will be in the same position as you would be in if you waited for a bus that isn't on the timetable when you think it absolutely should be. You will wait and wait and wait fruitlessly for a bus that will never come. The bald fact is this: confidence is not on the timetable when you begin to act in a self-disciplined way after years of self-undisciplined behaviour. Unconfidence is!

It is fine to hold a flexible belief about confidence in relation to engaging with a self-disciplined task. Thus, believing that it would be preferable but not essential to feel confident before engaging with the task is true: you do prefer to feel confident. It is also true that you don't have to feel confident before you act. It is logical, since both parts of this belief lack rigidity and thus the non-rigid conclusion can be logically derived from the non-rigid desire. Finally, your flexible belief will allow you to work under undesirable conditions if it makes sense for you to do so. It is undesirable for you to engage with a self-disciplined task when you are not feeling confident. However, doing so is in your interests because it is the only way you are going to reach your goals.

Finally, in allowing you to engage with the task while feeling unconfident, your flexible belief will allow you to learn an important fact: that you will become confident if you engage with the task unconfidently and persist with it until you develop confidence.

Competence

'I must be competent at the task before I can do it'

This is a similar belief to the one discussed above (i.e. 'I need to feel confident before I do the task') and similar arguments apply, since there is a close relationship between competence and confidence. However, since the two are not the same (e.g. you can be confident without being competent, and if you have low self-esteem you can certainly be competent without an accompanying sense of confidence), I have chosen to devote a separate section to the demand for pre-action competence.

While it is possible for some people to have confidence that they can do a task that they have not done before (whether or not such confidence is misplaced), it is not possible for the same people to say that they have competence at that same task (unless the task is closely related to a task that they are competent at). They can say that they 'feel' competent at the task, but this is really a matter of confidence rather than demonstrated competence. You can only *demonstrate* competence, and you can only do that if you allow yourself to begin a task when you are not competent at it.

The demand for pre-action competence is rigid, and how to deal with it

It has been shown that in order to be unconsciously competent at something you have to go through a number of stages first. Thus:

- *Stage 1*: unconscious incompetence
- *Stage 2*: conscious incompetence
- *Stage 3*: conscious competence
- *Stage 4*: unconscious competence.

When you are in a state of unconscious incompetence, you don't know what you don't know. When you discover what you don't know, you are in a state of conscious incompetence. At this point you need to learn and practise relevant skills in order to achieve the state of conscious competence where you still have to consciously think about what to do. Repeatedly practising these skills consciously will then help you to become competent without conscious thought. Only at this point have you reached the state of unconscious competence.

This model explains why the demand for pre-action competence is so unrealistic. It tells you that you have to be at Stage 3 before you engage with the self-disciplined task, whereas in reality you will be at either Stage 1 or Stage 2. If you accept this fact without liking it and go through the four stages, you will develop unconscious competence and this will help you to develop and sustain self-discipline.

Certainty

'I have to know what will happen if I carry out the self-disciplined task before I start it'

A demand for pre-action certainty comes in two major forms. In its first form, you believe that you must know what is going to happen before you act, whether the outcome is good or bad. In its second form, you believe that you must know that a bad outcome will *not* occur before you take self-disciplined action. Either way, if you hold a demand for pre-action certainty, it is certain that you will not take action because such pre-action certainty is impossible to have.

The demand for pre-action certainty is rigid, and how to deal with it

The demand for pre-action certainty is rigid because it means that you will not engage in the self-disciplined task until you know for sure what will happen or until you know for sure that bad things will not happen as a result of your engagement with this task. If you believe in a demand for pre-action certainty, you will engage in activities that are designed to gain such certainty rather than engage with the self-disciplined task. In doing so, you are displaying self-undisciplined behaviour since you are doing things that take you away from your major focus, which is the self-disciplined task.

As before, it is fine to hold a flexible belief about knowing the outcome of engaging in self-disciplined behaviour before you engage in it. Thus, believing that it would be preferable but not essential to have such certainty is true: you do prefer to have it; and it is also true that you don't have to have it to start the task. It is logical, since both parts of this belief lack rigidity and thus the non-rigid conclusion can be logically derived from the non-rigid desire. Finally, your flexible belief is helpful in that it will allow you to engage in the task when you lack such certainty. Here, when questioned you might say something like: 'Although I would like to know what will happen before I engage in the self-disciplined task, I acknowledge that I don't have to get what I want in this situation, and I also know that it is impossible to get such certainty. Thus, rather than engage in activities designed to achieve certainty, I will engage in the self-disciplined task instead because it will help me to achieve my goals, even though it is disappointing that my desire is not being met on this occasion.'

If you act on this flexible philosophy and do so repeatedly, and in particular if you refrain from seeking out certainty when it is not available to you, then you will learn to break the association between uncertainty and inaction. Instead, you will forge a new association between uncertainty and task-focused action.

External control

'I have to be in control of my environment before I begin my self-disciplined task'

Another pre-action condition that you may insist upon before engaging with the self-disciplined task is control. There are two types of control that you may demand: external control and internal control. I will discuss the first in this section and the second in the following section.

The demand for pre-action external control is rigid

By external control I mean the idea that you have a sense of being in charge of relevant conditions that are external to you. When you demand control over external conditions before you engage with your self-disciplined task, you are at the mercy of these conditions when you are not in a position to change them.

For example, Pete wanted to improve his muscle tone and went to the gym three times per week to work out. He also did daily exercise at home. His next door neighbour played music loudly and refused to turn it down when requested to by Pete, who found it very difficult to do his exercises when the music was playing. You may think that Pete was demanding the absence of noise before he started his exercises, but you would be wrong. In the course of trying to help Pete and myself understand the important ingredient here, Pete said the following: 'I think that if I knew that my neighbour would turn the music down if I asked him to then I would not be bothered about the noise. What really bothers me is the idea that he won't turn it down even if I ask him to. I just feel helpless!'

Notice two things here that are clues to the presence of a demand for external control. First, Pete is bothered by the noise only when he knows that he is not in control of it. As he says, if he knows that his neighbour *would* turn the music down, then he could do his exercises. So it is not the noise *per se* that in his mind stops him from engaging with his self-disciplined task. It is the sense that he is not in control. The fact that he does not exercise when he is not in control of this external condition shows that his belief is rigid. If he held a flexible preference for pre-action external control, he would exercise even though he held no control over his neighbour's noise. Pete's preference would be to have control over this external condition before exercising, but he would also acknowledge that he doesn't need such control in order to exercise. If he acted on this flexible preference, he would exercise whether or not he had control over his neighbour's noise.

Second, Pete says that he feels helpless when he can't control his neighbour's noise. People who demand external control often report experiencing helplessness when they are not in control of outside factors, and demand that they absolutely should have such control.

How to deal with your demand for pre-action external control

So what can you do if you have a demand for pre-action external control?

1 First, see that this demand is false, illogical and unhelpful.
2 Second, see that your alternative flexible preference for pre-action control is true, logical and helpful. (I have explained both of these points before in this chapter: see pp. 54–5.)
3 Then consider the wisdom of the first four lines of the Serenity Prayer by Reinhold Niebuhr:

> God grant me the serenity
> to accept the things I cannot change;
> courage to change the things I can;
> and wisdom to know the difference.

which I have adapted for the issue of external control:

God grant me the serenity
to accept the aspects outside of me that I cannot control;
courage to influence the aspects outside of me that I can control;
and wisdom to know the difference.

In reflecting on this reformulation of the Serenity Prayer, notice one important point. The real control that you have when faced with situations that are beyond your external control is rooted in your attitude of acceptance that appears in both the original Serenity Prayer and my reformulation of it. Since 'acceptance' is a word that has several meanings, in the next point I will spend a little time discussing it, as it is important that you understand the way that I employ the term.

4   Accept what you can't control. When you accept an aspect outside you that you can't control, you acknowledge the following:

- that the reality is that you are not able to control this aspect;
- that you prefer to have such external control, but that you do not need to have it;
- that it is unfortunate that you do not have such external control, but that it is not the end of the world that you don't have it;
- that it is uncomfortable that you don't have the control to change the external condition, but it is tolerable and worth tolerating;
- that it is important that you act on these beliefs. Thus, engage with the self-disciplined task that you previously avoided because you thought you needed pre-action external control. Refrain from acting to gain such external control even if your thoughts direct you to do so. Acknowledge that such thoughts are best left alone to be (as it were) and should not be acted on.

5   Finally, realize that you are not helpless. When you think that you are helpless in the face of being unable to control a relevant aspect of your environment, recognize that such a conclusion stems from your demand for pre-action external control. Working to change this demand will help, but you can also show yourself that while you are helpless in this one respect, you are not helpless overall. Don't forget that it is possible to change your attitude when you are faced with an environment that you can't control, and changing your attitude is a powerful antidote to generalized helplessness. Reflect on these wise and powerful words from Viktor Frankl (1905–97), author, neurologist, psychiatrist and Holocaust survivor:

We who lived in concentration camps can remember the men who walked through the huts comforting others, giving away their last piece of bread. They may have been few in number, but they offer sufficient proof that everything can be taken from a man but one thing: the last of the human freedoms – to choose one's attitude in any given set of circumstances, to choose one's own way.

Self-control

'I must be in control of myself before I take action'

This belief can refer to a range of experiences, all of which are internal to the person. Here is a selection of what people may demand that they have control over before they begin acting in a self-disciplined manner:

- their feelings
- their thoughts (including images)
- their urges
- their behaviour.

All this comes under the heading of a demand for pre-action self-control.

The demand for pre-action self-control is rigid

There are many drawbacks to a demand for pre-action self-control. Let's take the example of Brenda, an HR manager, whose goal was to become a trainer of HR personnel, a job that involved a lot of public speaking. Consequently, she resolved to become proficient at speaking in public in order to be qualified for this job. However, Brenda was anxious about speaking in public and, what is particularly relevant to our present discussion, she demanded that she must not be anxious before she gave presentations. As a result, she refused to do any public talks until she wasn't anxious about doing so. The problems with taking this stance are as follows:

1 Brenda's demand that she must be in control over her feelings so that she is not anxious means that the prospect of being anxious constitutes a threat to her, and since she is trying to eradicate her anxiety, this means that she becomes anxious about the possibility of being anxious. She thus perpetuates her problem.
2 Avoiding giving public talks means that Brenda never confronts her anxiety about feeling anxious.
3 By actually avoiding feeling anxiously out of control, Brenda unwittingly reinforces the idea that she has to avoid such feelings at all costs.

How to deal with your demand for pre-action self-control

So what can you do if you have a demand for pre-action self-control?

1 Once again, see that this demand is false, illogical and unhelpful.
2 Then, as before, acknowledge that your alternative flexible preference for pre-action self-control is true, logical and helpful. (I have explained both of these points before in this chapter; see pp. 54–5.)
3 Recognize that the best way to deal with your fear about not being in control is to experience this feeling while accepting but not liking it, and tolerating it. If you do this a number of times then you will begin to see that not being in control is uncomfortable, but not dangerous. You only think it is dangerous because by demanding that you have to be in control, you use only two categories: (a) in control and (b) out of control. By being flexible about not being in self-control, you are much more likely to understand and apply the idea that self-control is best placed on a continuum and that if you lose control of yourself a little, it does not mean that you are about to lose complete control of yourself. The fear of complete loss of self-control is produced by the demand for self-control.
4 It is very important that you act on your flexible preference for pre-action self-control. This means engaging with your self-disciplined task even though you are not in full self-control. If you repeatedly do this, you will overcome this obstacle to self-discipline.

Control and certainty

'I must know now that I will be in control later. Once I know that, then I will engage in my self-disciplined task'

In my 30 years' experience as a counsellor, I have discovered that the themes of control and certainty often go together in people's problems. When they do and they serve as an obstacle to self-disciplined action, the resultant belief is a variant of: 'I must know now that I will be in control later. Once I know that, then I will engage in my self-disciplined task.'

The demand for pre-action certainty and control is rigid

When you believe the above, you actually have two rigid beliefs which are closely linked together. First, you believe that you have to be in control (whether this refers to external or internal control), and second, you believe that you have to have certainty now that you will be in control at some point in the future. Demanding pre-action certainty and control means that you have erected a very powerful obstacle to self-disciplined action. For how are you to engage in a self-disciplined task which will invariably be accompanied by uncertainty and often by a sense that you may not be in full control, when you demand that you have to know now something that you can't possibly know? The answer is, you can't.

How to deal with your demand for pre-action certainty and control

As with other demands, it is important to recognize that your desire for pre-action certainty and control is OK as long as you recognize (1) that you don't have to have this desire met and (2) that you cannot have it met. Then it is important to engage with the self-disciplined task in the face of lack of certainty about later control and repeat this until it becomes second nature to you. As you act in a self-disciplined manner in the face of control-related uncertainty, be aware that you will still get thoughts and urges, the purpose of which is to try and get such certainty. This is coming from your STS and is quite usual. The important thing is to accept (without liking) the existence of these thoughts and urges and to refrain from acting on them. Continue to act in the service of your longer-term self-discipline goals.

Full comprehension

'I must understand all relevant parts of the task and the process before I take self-disciplined action'

While the need to fully understand is linked to the need for certainty, it is sufficiently different to merit separate consideration. Thus, if you believe that you have to understand a task fully before you do it, then you will do it if you have such understanding even if you lack certainty about what will happen if you do it. The important thing with this demand is that you believe that you must have full comprehension of what is involved in the task itself and in the process which links the task with your self-discipline goals.

The demand for pre-action full comprehension is rigid

As with other demands, the demand for pre-action full comprehension is rigid and virtually eliminates your capacity for self-disciplined action when you are faced with lack of understanding. If you hold such a belief, then you will spend an inordinate amount of time researching aspects of the self-disciplined task and the associated process rather than getting down to the task itself. For example, Jake had a dissertation to do for his undergraduate degree, and the effects of his demand for pre-action full comprehension were as follows:

• He collected all relevant articles to do with his project and read them all. While this may seem sensible, the extent of his research would have been more appropriate if Jake was doing a PhD. Over-researching an area is a typical effect of a demand for pre-action comprehension.

- He read many books on the process of carrying out a dissertation. Now, some research into this process is good practice, but Jake read far more books on this subject than was helpful, and indeed, he became confused by the contradictory advice he got from these books. People with a demand for pre-action comprehension are often intolerant of differing views on the same issue. They often seek the 'right' answer.
- Jake repeatedly went to his dissertation supervisor for help on his dissertation and on the process of writing one. Again, asking for some help is sensible, but doing it very often is a sign of comprehension-demand based insecurity. Such students are often experienced as 'high maintenance' by college tutors.

How to deal with your demand for pre-action comprehension

By now you should know that the first stage in dealing with any demand is to see that it is false, illogical and unhelpful to you. In contrast, your flexible alternative belief is true, logical and helpful. Thus, if you demand pre-action full comprehension you are ruling out the possibility of engaging with your self-disciplined task when you have some, but incomplete, understanding of what you have to do. As this possibility exists, your demand is false. Indeed, you will learn more about the task and the process of acquiring self-discipline through the experience of doing the task than if you research it through books (such as this one!) or by talking to people about their experiences of (a) doing the task and of (b) going through the process of developing self-discipline. Thus, your demand for pre-action full comprehension actually robs you of the best forum for learning, i.e. from your own experience. It is thus illogical and unhelpful.

By contrast, your flexible preference for pre-action full comprehension will help you to gain sufficient understanding to begin the task and will help you to learn 'on the job', as it were. While you may want pre-action full comprehension, it is also important not to act on this desire, since even your desire may lead you to be inefficient in encouraging you to spend too much time on second-hand learning, instead of learning experientially first-hand about the task and the process of developing self-discipline on the go.

If you hold a flexible preference about pre-action full comprehension, you will react to pre-action lack of understanding as a cue to begin the task rather than a cue to do more research. You will remind yourself that you don't need to know everything and that at this stage you probably know all you need to do the task.

Also, while it is good to know something of the process of developing self-discipline, your flexible preference for pre-action full comprehension will allow you to focus on the 'doing' of the self-disciplined task rather than on the 'how' of the process of becoming self-disciplined. Thus, your flexible preference for pre-action full comprehension allows you to be honest with yourself about what you want, encourages you to be realistic about what you can know and what you can't, and prompts you to engage with the self-disciplined task free from the shackles of having to know everything before you start.

Comfort

'I must be comfortable before I start the task'

Perhaps the most pernicious idea that you can hold in the field of self-discipline, that serves as a major obstacle to you in your quest to develop self-discipline, is the demand for pre-action comfort. I include here the demand for pre-action lack of discomfort.

The demand for pre-action comfort is rigid

If you demand pre-action comfort, the following is a common scenario. You have resolved to engage in a self-disciplined task, and as you approach doing it you start to feel uncomfortable. You then don't engage with the task because you are uncomfortable and you believe that you have to feel comfortable before starting the task. So you do something to make yourself comfortable, and when you have achieved a sense of comfort you approach the task again, only to feel uncomfortable again. So you back away from doing the task and seek comfort. As you do this you are sowing the seeds for a self-defeating pattern where, because of your demand for pre-action comfort, you teach yourself to respond to discomfort with avoidance. Because you are rigid about comfort, you do not have the flexibility to engage with your self-disciplined task when you are uncomfortable.

How to deal with your demand for pre-action comfort

As with other demands, you need to see that the demand for pre-action comfort is:

- false (you *can* act while feeling uncomfortable);
- illogical (you may want to feel comfortable before you act, but it does not follow that you have to do so); and
- unhelpful (you will only engage with the self-disciplined task when you are comfortable).

Then, you need to see that your preference for pre-action comfort is

- true (it is true that you want to be comfortable before you act and it is also true that you don't have to have such comfort before starting);
- logical (you want to be comfortable before you act, and it logically follows that you don't have to be so); and
- helpful (you can engage with the self-disciplined task whether you are comfortable or not).

This belief change work will only help you if you act in ways that are consistent with your flexible preference for comfort and refrain from acting in ways that are consistent with your rigid demand. This means, in effect, that you need to engage with your self-disciplined task at designated times whether you feel comfortable or not. Indeed, if you are to strengthen your flexible preference, it is best if you engage with your self-disciplined task when you are feeling uncomfortable. If you do this, you practise the idea that you don't have to feel comfortable when you are feeling uncomfortable.

Also, you need to accept that your STS will frequently urge you to seek out comfort when you are experiencing discomfort. When this happens, show yourself that you don't need to go for immediate comfort, keep engaged with the self-disciplined task when you are feeling uncomfortable and, if necessary, review the reasons you are choosing to take a long-term perspective and why it is in your interest to tolerate the discomfort rather than alleviate it. Remember that if you tolerate discomfort, it will initially increase and then decrease if you stay engaged with the self-disciplined task.

You also need to accept that even though you have not responded to the promptings of your STS's need for immediate comfort, it will keep urging you to satisfy it. When this happens, all you need to do is to continue with the task and not respond to these urgings. Don't ignore them, because this implies an act of will which may well mean that you become more aware of the 'voice' of your STS. Why? Because ignoring this voice, not thinking about it, putting it out of your mind and distracting yourself from it are all designed to silence the voice of your STS. If this is your goal and you fail to achieve it, which I argue you invariably will, you will become discouraged and silence your STS in the only reliable way you know – by giving it what it wants.

Since silencing the STS in productive ways will not work, you need a different strategy. This strategy involves you doing the following:

- Accept the existence of the continuing voice of the STS and do not engage with it (after the initial challenge of the demand for comfort which underpins it). The STS is not interested in listening to reason. It is only interested in having what it sees as its needs satisfied, and it will respond to your reasoned arguments with all kinds of illogical arguments. If you engage with the STS and try to respond to these arguments (after your initial challenge of the STS's 'need' for comfort) then you will stop focusing on the task and get diverted into a fruitless quest to silence the voice of your STS – this time through reason. This is what the STS wants, since it knows it won't be silenced other than by the gratification of its 'need' for comfort. It hopes that you will eventually give in and gratify it. Stopping your work on the self-disciplined task to engage the STS in a logical argument increases the chances that the STS will get what it wants!

- While accepting the existence of the voice of your STS and not engaging with it, turn instead to the self-disciplined task and stay engaged with it while the STS is doing its best to derail you. Recognize that the STS is basically a spoiled child. Such a child is used to getting its own way. It has learned that if it nags you to satisfy its urges then you will give in to it. So when you don't respond in the accustomed way it thinks: 'Oh, perhaps you haven't heard me. I will make my voice stronger.' This is why, when you don't satisfy your STS, it will increase the number and intensity of its promptings. It needs to learn by experience – and not by reason – that you will not respond to it. So recognize that it is very important that you continue working on your self-disciplined task while the STS is doing its best to tempt you. Do not, I repeat, do not stop and respond in any way to your STS at this stage. Eventually, it will learn that its old way of getting what it wants will not work. Yes, it will try again next time, but your goal is to teach it that it will not get its 'needs' met under these conditions and you do this by not engaging with it after the initial challenge. What you are effectively doing here is challenging your demand for pre-action comfort by acting in ways that are inconsistent with the demand and acting in ways that are consistent with your flexible preference. In this way you increase the chances that you and your STS will learn that you do not, I repeat, do not have to feel comfortable before you begin a task.
- You need to repeat the above steps every time you engage with the self-disciplined task.

How to deal with your demand for comfort during the task

While I have focused on helping you deal with your demand for *pre-action* comfort, the same principles apply if you hold a demand for comfort *during* the execution of your self-disciplined task. Thus, if you begin to feel uncomfortable halfway through the task and it is not time for a brief scheduled break, then persist with the task even though you are feeling uncomfortable. Remember that, if you do this, your level of discomfort will increase in the short term, but will go down if you stay focused on the task. Also, when you deal with your demand for comfort while you are engaged in the task, anticipate that your STS will try to tempt you to seek immediate comfort when you are feeling uncomfortable during task engagement and will increase the number and intensity of its arguments if you do not engage with it. However, if you stay task-focused and do not engage with your STS, it will eventually get the message that you are not going to satisfy it and you will be able to continue with the task without due interruption from your STS.

Favourable external conditions

'Favourable external conditions must be present before I begin the self-disciplined task'

In one sense all the pre-action demanded conditions that I have discussed so far in this chapter are experiential and internal to the person making the demand. By experiential, I mean that the person is seeking an experience of comfort, control, certainty, etc. When people don't achieve the experiential sense of being comfortable, in control, certain, etc., then their demand impels them to keep demanding this experiential sense. Paradoxically, in their desperation to achieve the demanded sense, they often achieve the opposite. Thus, if you demand comfort and immediate comfort is not to hand, then desperately seeking comfort will make you more uncomfortable. If you feel out of control and you desperately seek the sense of being in control, you will more often than not feel more out of control.

However, not all pre-action demanded conditions are internal. Some are decidedly external, and in this final section of the chapter I will discuss demands for pre-action favourable external conditions and how to deal with them.

To illustrate what I mean, let me discuss two people who demanded the existence of favourable external conditions before engaging with self-disciplined tasks.

The demand for pre-action tidiness and how to deal with it

Laura wanted to gain advancement in her career, and she was told by her boss that her promotion depended on her doing a good job on the Lucas report. She resolved to do a good job, but kept putting off her work in favour of tidying her office. Laura believed that her office had to be tidy before she started to work. If her office was not tidy, she argued, she could not concentrate on her work. I helped Laura to:

1 see that wanting a tidy office before she started work was fine, but

it didn't follow that this favourable external condition had to be present in order for Laura to work;

2 understand that the only way she would truly grasp this point was to act on it. Thus, I encouraged Laura to begin work without first tidying her office. I helped her to accept she would still have the urge to tidy her office before she started work. Letting the urges be present while working on the Lucas report was particularly helpful to her in learning that she didn't have to act on her urges.

The demand for pre-action quiet and how to deal with it

Barry believed that he had to have perfect silence before meditating. As a result, he found it very difficult to find an environment where he could meditate. Even when he did occasionally find such a quiet place, he still found meditation difficult because he was anxious in case his quiet was interrupted by noise. I helped Barry to:

1 see that wanting a quiet environment before he meditated would cause Barry no problem as long as he also recognized that such a favourable external condition was not essential for this activity;

2 understand that one of the main purposes of meditation is to focus on something like a mantra while accepting external and internal disruptions to this focus. Thus, demanding a quiet environment in which to meditate may actually hinder Barry from learning how to maintain his attentional focus in the face of an external disruption.

Consequently, Barry looked for a relatively quiet environment in which to meditate rather than a perfectly quiet one, and as a result was able to meditate every day and get the benefit from it.

In the next chapter, I will show you how you can capitalize on your planning for self-disciplined action and on the work you have done dealing with the potential obstacles to such action.

7

Act in a self-disciplined manner

A famous writer was once asked what was the secret of writing. He thought for a moment and then said: 'The secret of writing is putting the seat of your pants on the seat of the chair and ... writing!' Although this sounds flippant it has a simple truth at its core. So, when I am asked for the secret of self-discipline, I take a leaf out of the writer's book and reply: 'The secret of self-discipline is taking action that is in your considered healthy interests, no matter how you feel, within reason.'

If you 'deconstruct' this phrase you will see that it comprises three elements:

- taking action
- the healthy purpose of the action
- the conditions for action.

I discussed the issue of the purpose of self-disciplined action in Chapter 1, and in Chapter 6 I showed you how to respond to the conditions that you think must exist before you engage in self-disciplined behaviour. In this chapter, I will focus on issues to do with taking action.

Take action

From one perspective, all one can say about taking action can be summed up in the Nike slogan: 'Just do it.' This actually has a great appeal because it is possible to over-analyse the process of taking action. Indeed, one of the obstacles that may prevent you from taking self-disciplined action may be your belief that you need to understand what you are going to do before you do it (see Chapter 6). From another perspective, however, taking action is not as simple as it sounds and raises certain issues that I am going to consider here.

Start

In my counselling practice, I deal with many clients who have problems with self-discipline. In listening to these people describe their difficulties, I have learned that most of them have problems with starting a self-disciplined task.

My sense is that at the root of this problem is the difficulty people experience making the transition from a current (often comfortable) state to a state of discomfort that almost inevitably accompanies initiating a self-disciplined task.

It follows from this (as I discussed in Chapter 6) that you increase the chances of initiating a self-disciplined task the fewer conditions you insist have to exist before starting it. So, if I were to change the Nike slogan, I would change it to: 'Do it uncomfortably.' If you begin a self-disciplined task uncomfortably, you will experience an initial increase in these feelings of discomfort which will then soon decrease if you continue with the task. Part of the problem with starting a task and the associated discomfort of doing so is that you often overestimate how uncomfortable you will feel on starting the task and how long you will experience this discomfort. Rather than put these hunches to the test, which is what you need to do, you think that your hunches are reality and thus don't start the task in order to spare yourself the experience of great long-lasting discomfort. Since you don't start the task, as I have said, you do not get the experience of the discomfort reducing quite quickly.

Use chunking

When you choose to act in a self-disciplined way and the task is complex or extended, you are faced with two questions:

- What does the task comprise? (which I dealt with in Chapter 5)
- How do I best divide up the doing of the task?

The second question is different from the question of how much time you are going to devote to task-related work in any one sitting, although it is related to it. You can look at a sub-task and further divide it in a way that makes sense to you and/or is manageable in that sitting. Then you can allocate time to that chunk of work. When I am in writing mode, I set myself a target of writing 500 words a day and I devote as much time as I need to achieve this goal. Also, I tend not to write this number of words in one sitting. I would say I achieve this writing target on average in three small 'writing chunks'. Alternatively, you can use time as the chunk and do as much work as you can in that time period.

The point that I want to emphasize here is that it is important that you choose the chunking method that best facilitates your self-disciplined task behaviour.

Colin's example
Colin set as his self-discipline goal to do his essays on time. He then looked closely at the particular essay that he had to write and divided it into its component parts. I showed how he did this in Chapter 5. Colin then took each component and decided to write in two-hour chunks first thing in the morning, as outlined in the preparation and planning section (pp. 49–52). He actually did this with the help of some

belief-change statements that challenged the idea that he had to be comfortable before he started.

Take sensible breaks

People differ as to how much they can concentrate on a complex task in one sitting. In addition, different tasks require different levels of concentration. As a result, you need to consider your self-disciplined task and take sensible breaks when appropriate. The purpose of a break is to refresh and rejuvenate you so that you come back to the task with renewed mental and/or physical energy. As such, I suggest that you regard any other reason for taking a break (other than to deal with an emergency) as self-undisciplined behaviour. Thus, when you take a break because you are feeling very uncomfortable or you are stuck, then you are avoiding the task and are acting in a self-undisciplined way. If you are feeling uncomfortable, then stay with the discomfort and you will find that it fades away gradually. If you are stuck and you accept the stuckness, then doing so will help you to move forward.

Colin's example
As we have recalled, Colin decided to work on his essay in two-hour chunks, first thing in the morning. He decided to take two ten-minute coffee breaks in that time period. This helped to sustain him for the entire two-hour sitting.

Restart

If you take a planned break from self-disciplined behaviour or stop for any other reason (e.g. to answer the front door or to go to the toilet), then it is important that you restart the task immediately. As I discussed above, moving from the state of 'not carrying out the task' to the state of 'carrying out the task' may be difficult for you, particularly if you believe that you have to be comfortable before you start or restart the task. This is what I call 'transition discomfort'. If restarting the task is a problem for you, it is important that you act on the idea that you can restart the task while feeling uncomfortable and that it is worth it to you to do so. If necessary, rehearse it in your mind or, if it is practicable, speak it out loud (e.g. 'I can continue with the task even though I may well experience discomfort'), which is what Colin did after coming back from his coffee breaks.

Stop when it is healthy to do so

I mentioned earlier that it is useful to carry out self-disciplined behaviour in manageable chunks, where these chunks are defined by time (e.g. in Colin's case, two hours) or by a set amount of the task (e.g. in my case 500 words per day). Once you have got into the task, you may find it difficult to stop. Stopping may lead you to experience a somewhat different form of transition discomfort where this time the discomfort you experience occurs when you move from the state of 'carrying out the task' to the state of 'not carrying out the task'.

You may think that experiencing difficulty in stopping self-disciplined behaviour when you have nominated to do so is a blessing, not a curse, and to some degree you may be right, so long as you do stop soon after you have achieved your daily self-disciplined target. However, if you go on for too long you may create additional problems for yourself. Thus, you may:

- overtire yourself;
- lose sleep;
- become stale;
- become obsessed;
- miss out on pleasurable activities.

A common form of difficulty stopping a self-disciplined task once you have started it occurs when you believe that you have to finish the task in one sitting. As a result you refuse to go to bed, for example, until you have finished the task. To deal with this problem you do need to access that part of you that I have called the 'executive self', that part of you that is concerned, among other things, with helping you to have balance in your life. You need to learn that life is more enjoyable when you have a balance between fun and self-discipline. Consequently, you need to tolerate the discomfort of stopping and practise the healthy idea that you don't have to finish any self-disciplined task in one go, particularly when in doing so you harm yourself in ways that I mentioned above.

Colin's example
Colin did not experience a problem with stopping self-disciplined behaviour once he had completed his nominated two hours of essay writing.

This concludes my discussion of self-discipline that involves taking action. In the next part of the book, I will discuss self-discipline that involves refraining from taking self-undisciplined action.

Part 4

When self-discipline involves refraining from taking self-undisciplined action

In the previous part of the book, I discussed the type of self-discipline that involves taking disciplined action and illustrated my points with reference to the example of Colin, whose self-disciplined behavioural target was working on his essay. In this part of the book, I will discuss self-discipline which involves refraining from taking self-undisciplined action and illustrate my points with respect to the example of Glenda, whose self-disciplined behavioural target was refraining from smoking.

8

Plan and prepare to refrain from self-undisciplined behaviour

If your target is to develop self-discipline that involves refraining from taking self-undisciplined action, you also need to make effective plans and properly prepare yourself in order to maximize the chances that you will develop this type of self-discipline. If you rely on your ability in the moment to act in a self-disciplined manner without proper planning and preparation, two things will happen. You will increase the chances that you will continue to act in a self-undisciplined way and decrease your chances of developing what I will henceforth call 'refraining-based' self-discipline.

The following are important elements to such effective planning and preparation.

Anticipating external cues to self-undisciplined behaviour

If your goal is to refrain from acting in a self-undisciplined manner, then an important part of your preparation will be to understand the cues to which you typically respond with that behaviour. The purpose of such understanding is to help you to anticipate such cues and triggers so that you deal with them effectively and do not act in a self-undisciplined way.

As I have already stated, this book is partly based on the ideas of Rational Emotive Behaviour Therapy (REBT), a specific form of cognitive behaviour therapy (CBT) developed by the American clinical psychologist Albert Ellis in 1955. One of the basic tenets of CBT is that a situation provides the context for your self-undisciplined behaviour, but it does not trigger it. According to CBT, it is the thoughts you have in the situation that are largely responsible for triggering your self-undisciplined behaviour, not the situation itself. For this reason, I distinguish between external cues to self-undisciplined behaviour and internal triggers of that same behaviour.

In this part of the chapter, I will briefly consider the external cues, but will concentrate more on the internal triggers. My purpose in doing so is twofold. First, I have already considered the external cues to self-undisciplined behaviour in Chapter 4. Second, as the REBT model holds, dealing with internal triggers to self-undisciplined behaviour is more important than dealing with external cues, since the former rather than the latter are the prime determinants of such behaviour.

External cues

An external cue to self-undisciplined behaviour is, as the term implies, a cue that is external to you as a person. In Chapter 4, I suggested that it is important for you to monitor your self-undisciplined behaviour and suggested a formal way of doing this, as shown in the box.

Date	Time	Situation	Alone/with others	Description of self-undisciplined behaviour

When you monitor your self-undisciplined behaviour using the form presented in Appendix 2, you will be able to identify recurring patterns in the external cues to which you respond with that behaviour. I suggest that you review Chapter 4 if you need to refresh your memory of the points in that chapter.

Let me bring that material to life by reconsidering the example of Ellen, whom we first met in Chapter 4. Ellen targeted overeating as the self-undisciplined behaviour that she wished to address. In particular, her goal was to eat three good meals a day and not to eat between meals. As I showed in Chapter 4, Ellen's monitoring form indicated two patterns. She overeats (1) when she is alone in her kitchen (here she eats savoury foodstuffs) and (2) when she is watching TV in the lounge with David, her partner (here she eats chocolate bars).

Identifying the internal triggers to self-undisciplined behaviour

As I have said, dealing effectively with internal triggers to self-undisciplined behaviour is central to developing self-discipline, and therefore it is crucial that you adequately prepare yourself to deal with your internal triggers.

In order to do this, you need to incorporate internal triggers into the self-monitoring framework reproduced in Appendix 2. In doing so, we need a sixth heading – 'Thinking' – which is best placed just before the heading 'Description of self-undisciplined behaviour' to emphasize that thinking largely triggers self-undisciplined behaviour. Thus:

Date	Time	Situation	Alone/with others	Thinking	Description of self-undisciplined behaviour

As I have just noted, this book is partly based on REBT. This form of CBT places particular emphasis on the impact of rigid and extreme beliefs on emotions and behaviour. I outlined this approach in Chapter 2. It is a very important part of your planning and preparing to develop refraining-based self-discipline that you understand the role of rigid and extreme beliefs in triggering self-undisciplined behaviour. Consequently, I suggest that, if you need to, you review the material in Chapter 2 before proceeding with this chapter.

Rigid beliefs vs. flexible beliefs

As I explained in Chapter 2, both rigid and flexible beliefs are usually based on your desires and preferences. These indicate what you want to happen and what you don't want to happen. When your beliefs are rigid, you demand that your preferences are met and these encourage you to act in self-undisciplined ways. When your beliefs are flexible, by contrast, you recognize that you don't have to get what you want in life, and as such these flexible beliefs will help you to refrain from acting in self-undisciplined ways.

Flexible beliefs

In REBT theory, flexible beliefs normally take the form of non-dogmatic preferences. Let's suppose that you have set giving up smoking as your self-discipline goal, and let's further assume that you hold the following flexible belief: 'When I am offered a cigarette, I want to feel the coolness of the taste in my mouth, but I don't have to have this experience.' The preference part of this belief: 'When I am offered a cigarette, I want to feel the coolness of the taste in my mouth ...' leads you to have the urge to accept a cigarette if it is offered to you. However, the second part of this belief (which I call the non-demanding part), where you acknowledge that you don't have to have this experience, encourages you to pause and not to immediately take a cigarette when it is offered to you. Having reflected on it, using your executive self (ES) you won't take the offered cigarette because you have set as your goal to develop greater self-discipline by refraining from smoking. Thus, the second part of the flexible belief allows you to engage your long-term self (LTS), and when you do this you markedly increase the chances that you will act in ways that are self-disciplined in nature.

As I explained in Chapter 2, note that non-dogmatic preferences have two components. In the first component (the 'asserted preference' component), you are asserting what you want or prefer to happen. In the second component (the 'negated demand' component) you are acknowledging that you don't have to have your preferences met. It is this latter component that makes such beliefs flexible.

Rigid beliefs

In REBT theory, rigid beliefs normally take the form of demands. What makes these demands rigid is the transformation of your preferences into demands. For example, again assume that you hold the preference first outlined above: 'When I am offered a cigarette, I want to feel the coolness of the taste in my mouth ...' If you make this belief rigid, you transform it thus: '... and therefore I have to have this experience.' Once again your preference leads you to have the urge to accept a cigarette when it is offered to you, and the rigid transformation almost guarantees that you will act on your urge and thus engage with the very self-undisciplined behaviour that you have targeted for change.

Thus, demands also have two components. The first (the 'asserted preference' component) is the same as in flexible, non-dogmatic preferences in that it asserts your preferences. In the second (the 'demand' component'), you insist that you have to have your preferences met. It is this latter transformation that makes such demands rigid.

While rigid demands are frequently based on preferences, as I have shown, they are more frequently stated without the preference part being made explicit, as can be seen here: 'When I am offered a cigarette, I have to have the experience of the cool taste in my mouth.'

As I have shown, what is most problematic about a rigid belief in the context of your attempts to develop refraining-based self-discipline is that it gives you no room to manoeuvre. Since you believe that you have to have the experience of the coolness of the taste of a cigarette, for example, you impel yourself to have this experience and thus you end up by acting in a self-undisciplined manner. I will show you how to respond to rigid beliefs in Chapter 9, but for now your goal is to identify their presence, since you are preparing yourself to refrain from engaging in self-undisciplined behaviour.

Extreme beliefs vs. non-extreme beliefs

As I explained in Chapter 2, the founder of REBT, Albert Ellis, has argued that three extreme beliefs stem from rigid beliefs. Thus, if you hold a rigid demand then the conclusions that you are likely to make are likely to be extreme in nature. The three extreme beliefs that stem from rigid beliefs are known in REBT as:

- awfulizing beliefs
- low frustration tolerance (LFT) beliefs, and
- depreciation beliefs.

Their healthy counterparts are known as:

- non-awfulizing beliefs
- high frustration tolerance (HFT) beliefs, and
- acceptance beliefs.

Like rigid beliefs, extreme beliefs tend to give you no room to manoeuvre and lead you to act in self-undisciplined ways because they allow you access to neither your ES nor your LTS. As they are extreme beliefs, they tend to come from your short-term self (STS), which urges you to rid yourself of the disturbed feelings – which stem from your extreme beliefs – by acting in self-undisciplined ways.

Like flexible beliefs, non-extreme beliefs tend to give you room to manoeuvre and lead you to act in self-disciplined ways because they allow you to access your ES and your LTS. The former allows you to think of how to satisfy your short-term desires without sabotaging your longer-term self-discipline goals, while the latter is concerned with how you can reach these longer-term goals. Also, as they are non-extreme, these beliefs are by no means dominated by your STS and thus you are more likely to stay with and respond effectively to the negative but non-disturbed feelings which occur when your flexible desires are unmet. This tolerance also helps you to achieve your longer-term goals through self-disciplined behaviour. I will discuss these beliefs one at a time and contrast them with their healthy non-extreme alternatives.

Awfulizing beliefs vs. non-awfulizing beliefs

These beliefs are concerned with appraisals about how bad an experience is. When you hold a rigid belief, for example, then your appraisals are likely to be extreme in nature. When you hold an awfulizing belief, you believe that it will be awful, terrible or the end of the world if you don't get what you demand. So, if you believe: 'When I am offered a cigarette, I have to have the experience of the cool taste in my mouth,' then you will tend to conclude: 'It will be awful not having the cool taste of the cigarette in my mouth.'

On the other hand, if your belief is flexible then your appraisals are likely to be non-extreme in nature. When you hold a non-awfulizing belief, you believe that it will be bad, but not awful, terrible or the end of the world if you don't get what you prefer but do not demand. So, if you believe: 'When I am offered a cigarette, I want to feel the coolness of the taste in my mouth, but I don't have to have this experience,' then you will tend to conclude 'It will be bad, but not awful, not having the cool taste of the cigarette in my mouth.'

There are two components of non-awfulizing beliefs.

1 In the first component (the 'asserted badness' component), you are

asserting that not getting what you want, but do not demand, is bad (how bad it is depends on how much you want it). Thus: 'It will be bad not having the taste of the cigarette in my mouth ...'

2 In the second component (the 'negated awfulizing' component), you are acknowledging that it is not awful if you don't get what you want. Thus: '... but it would not be awful not having this taste.'

Low frustration tolerance (LFT) beliefs vs. high frustration tolerance (HFT) beliefs

These beliefs are concerned with your judgement about how able you are to tolerate an experience. When you hold a rigid belief, for example, then your judgement in this respect will again be extreme. When you hold an LFT belief, you believe that it will be intolerable if you don't get what you demand. So, if you believe: 'When I am offered a cigarette, I have to have the experience of the cool taste in my mouth,' then you will tend to conclude: 'I couldn't bear not having the cool taste of the cigarette in my mouth.'

On the other hand, if your belief is flexible, then your judgement about how tolerable an experience is will be non-extreme. Thus, when you hold an HFT belief, you believe that it will be a struggle but tolerable if you don't get what you prefer but do not demand. So, if you believe: 'When I am offered a cigarette, I want to feel the coolness of the taste in my mouth, but I don't have to have this experience,' then you will tend to conclude: 'It will be difficult, but I can bear not having the cool taste of the cigarette in my mouth and it is worth it to me to do so.'

There are three components of HFT beliefs.

1 In the first component (the 'asserted struggle' component), you are asserting that when you are faced with an adversity, you find it difficult to put up with it. Thus: 'It will be difficult not having the cool taste of the cigarette in my mouth ...'

2 In the second component (the 'negated unbearability' component), you are acknowledging that you can put up with the adversity. Thus: '... but I can bear foregoing this taste ...'

3 Finally, in the third component (which I call the 'worth tolerating' component), you show yourself that it is worth tolerating the adversity if doing so leads to greater self-discipline. Thus: '... and it is worth it to me to do so.'

Depreciation beliefs vs. acceptance beliefs

These beliefs are concerned with your attitude to yourself, others and/ or life conditions. As I considered self-depreciation and self-acceptance in Chapter 3, I will focus here on other-depreciation/other-acceptance and life-depreciation/life-acceptance. When you hold a rigid belief, for example, your attitude towards others and life will be extreme in the sense that you tend to depreciate both others and life conditions. So, if you believe: 'When I am offered a cigarette, I have to have the experience of the cool taste in my mouth,' then you will tend to conclude: 'Life would be no good if I were to deprive myself of this taste.' This is an example of life-depreciation.

On the other hand, if your belief is flexible then your attitude towards others and life will be non-extreme, in the sense that you will tend to accept both others and life conditions even though they both have negative aspects. So, if you believe: 'When I am offered a cigarette, I want to feel the coolness of the taste in my mouth, but I don't have to have this experience,' then you will tend to conclude: 'If I deprive myself of this taste, this aspect of life is not good, but this does not mean that life is bad. Rather, life is a complex mixture of good, bad and neutral aspects.' This is an example of life-acceptance.

There are three components of acceptance beliefs as illustrated with a life-acceptance belief.

1 In the first component (the 'negatively evaluated aspect' component), you evaluate an aspect of life or another person when these aspects serve to frustrate you in some way. Thus: 'If I deprive myself of the cool taste of a cigarette, this aspect of life is not good ...'
2 In the second component (the 'negated global negative evaluation' component), you acknowledge that you cannot legitimately rate the whole of another person or rate life on the basis of one or more of their/its aspects. Thus: '... but that does not mean that life is bad ...'
3 In the third and final component (the 'asserted complex' component), you assert that life is complex. Thus: '... Rather, life itself is a complex mixture of good, bad and neutral aspects.'

Distinguishing between beliefs and automatic thoughts

Having outlined the rigid and extreme beliefs that underpin self-undisciplined behaviour, I will show you how to use this material to identify these unhelpful beliefs. If you recall, I suggested that you monitor your self-undisciplined behaviour using the following framework:

Date	Time	Situation	Alone/with others	Thinking	Description of self-undisciplined behaviour

When you complete the section on thinking, you need to ask yourself what was going through your mind at the time when you were acting in a self-undisciplined manner but your goal was to act in a self-disciplined manner. If you ask yourself this question then you will probably identify what are called automatic thoughts, to which you

Table 6 Ellen's example expanded

Date	Time	Situation	Alone/ with others	Thinking	Description of self-undisciplined behaviour
17/3	6.25 p.m.	Kitchen	Alone	I'm bored (*and I need cheering up now*)	Ate six slices of bread
17/3	7.12 p.m.	Kitchen	Alone	I feel empty (*and I can't bear this feeling*)	Ate five Cream Crackers
17/3	7.30 p.m.	Lounge	With David	I would like the taste of chocolate (*and it would be terrible not to have it*)	Ate one Mars bar watching TV
17/3	8.03 p.m.	Lounge	With David	It would be good to join David (*so I must be sociable*)	Ate half a Crunchie bar watching TV

need to add your unhelpful beliefs. Let me illustrate this by referring to Ellen's example in Table 6.

If we take Ellen's first entry, we see that she was in the kitchen on her own and she ended up eating six slices of bread, which she recognized later as being self-undisciplined behaviour. Now, let's closely examine her thinking. Her automatic thought (i.e. the thought that passed through her mind at the time she was eating the bread) was 'I'm bored.' However, according to REBT theory this automatic thought is not sufficient to explain Ellen's self-undisciplined eating. Not everybody who is bored overeats, for example. Rather, Ellen ate because she held a rigid idea that underpinned this automatic thought, namely, 'I need cheering up now.' Since Ellen believed that she needed to cheer herself up immediately, she looked around her environment and raided the cupboard, as she had learned (or rather taught herself) that eating foods from the cupboard put an immediate end to her feelings of boredom. However, it also put an immediate end to her disciplined eating regime! If we look at Ellen's other episodes where she failed to refrain from acting in a self-undisciplined manner we see the same principle at work:

Automatic thought	*Underlying unhealthy belief*
I am bored ...	... and I need cheering up.
I feel empty ...	... and I can't bear this feeling.
I would like the taste of chocolate ...	... and it would be terrible not to have it.
It would be good to join David ...	... and so I have to be sociable.

In identifying your unhelpful beliefs, I suggest that you follow these instructions:

- Identify what was going through your mind just before you acted in the self-undisciplined manner that you have targeted for change.
- Add to this automatic thought the major unhelpful belief that accounted for your failure to refrain from acting in a self-undisciplined manner. Choose one of the following that best accounted for your self-undisciplined behaviour:
  - a demand
  - an awfulizing belief
  - a LFT belief
  - a self/other or life-depreciation belief.

Alternatively, you can ask yourself the following questions:

- 'Just before I acted in a self-undisciplined way ...
  - What was I demanding?
  - What was I saying was awful?
  - What did I think I could not tolerate?
  - Was I depreciating myself/others or the world?'

Select the one unhelpful belief which best accounted for your self-undisciplined behaviour.

Once you have identified the main unhelpful belief, your next step is to question these beliefs and to develop healthy alternative beliefs. This is the subject of the next chapter, with special reference to dealing with urges to self-undisciplined behaviour. You can also prepare yourself in your quest to refrain from acting in a self-undisciplined way by developing, if relevant, a healthy alternative to this behaviour. I will now consider this issue.

Developing alternative behaviours

When you develop refraining-based self-discipline in this context you are actually doing two things. First, you are refraining from acting in ways that interfere with your healthy goals. Second, and less obviously, you are developing and practising what might be called a self-discipline philosophy, a set of helpful beliefs that underpin successful attempts to refrain from acting in self-undisciplined ways. Here is a succinct summary of this philosophy:

When I am faced with the option of acting in ways that are immediately satisfying or relieving to me but which are ultimately self-defeating, I do not have to take this option, even though I may strongly wish to in the moment. If I refrain from acting in such self-undisciplined ways then that is frustrating, but not terrible. It is difficult to tolerate such deprivation, but I can tolerate it and it is worth it to me to do so. Finally, while this may be an adversity for me, the world is not a bad place for not giving me ideal conditions (where I can have what I want without being penalized for doing so in the longer term).

Pitfalls

When you are working on refraining from engaging in self-undisciplined behaviour, it may be useful to develop a behavioural alternative to that behaviour, something you can engage in instead. While on the face of it this seems like a good idea, there are pitfalls to it and you need to understand these pitfalls before choosing such a behavioural alternative.

Not rehearsing the philosophy underpinning self-discipline

If you are considering a behaviour that might be a good alternative to the self-undisciplined behaviour from which you wish to refrain, then it is important to make sure that you give yourself the opportunity of practising a relevant version of the above philosophy before you carry out this behaviour.

For example, Glenda (whom we first met in Chapter 4) set as her goal refraining from smoking. She found it particularly difficult to refuse taking a cigarette when offered one by one of her 'smoking group' when out for a drink. To help herself, Glenda decided to do the following when someone offered her a cigarette in this context. She would say 'no' and immediately phone one of her non-smoking friends for support and encouragement. While this may sound like a good solution to dealing with temptation, the important point is that if she takes this tack she will not practise her self-discipline philosophy. Indeed, she will be unwittingly practising the following beliefs that underpin her self-undisciplined behaviour:

- 'I can't stand the discomfort of depriving myself of a cigarette and need to distract myself from this discomfort.'
- 'I can't do this alone and need others to help me.'

Ideally, in order to avoid reinforcing these unhelpful beliefs, Glenda needs to tolerate the discomfort involved with not taking the cigarette. She needs to gain the experience of noticing her discomfort level falling after initially rising when she refrains from smoking. In this way, she can learn that she does not have to distract herself from discomfort in order to deal with it productively. Once she has tolerated the discomfort associated with deprivation, then, if she thinks that calling her friend for support and encouragement will help her further, that would be the time to make the call.

Engaging in other self-undisciplined behaviours

One of the biggest obstacles to developing refraining-based self-discipline is engaging in another form of self-undisciplined behaviour instead. A common form of this phenomenon was shown by Glenda in a previous attempt to give up smoking. In the past, whenever she experienced an urge to smoke, Glenda ate something instead, with the result that although she gave up smoking she put on a lot of weight. As she found being overweight more problematic than not smoking, Glenda went back to smoking in order to lose weight.

One of the main reasons people replace one self-undisciplined behaviour with another is that they have not addressed the unhelpful beliefs that underpin their lack of self-discipline. In particular, the philosophy of low frustration tolerance (LFT) is often involved when a person engages in one form of self-undisciplined behaviour to cope with refraining from engaging with the target self-undisciplined behaviour. This can be clearly shown in Glenda's reply when I interviewed her on her past attempts at giving up smoking. In response to my questions concerning her use of food to help her give up smoking, Glenda said that whenever she refrained from smoking when she wanted a cigarette, she felt very uncomfortable, accompanied by a strong urge to have a cigarette. In order to cope with the urge to smoke and the discomfort of deprivation, Glenda turned to food and did so as soon as she began to have these two experiences. One of the tell-tale signs that a person is operating according to a philosophy of LFT in this context is the speed with which that person switches to another form of self-undisciplined behaviour. The quicker the switch, the more likely the presence of an LFT philosophy.

If Glenda could have articulated her LFT belief at the time she would have said something like this:

> I can't stand the discomfort of not having a cigarette when I want one and I have to get rid of the urge to have one. In order to get rid of both the discomfort and the urge as quickly as possible, I will satisfy myself by eating chocolate. If I don't do that then my feelings of discomfort and the urge will grow to intolerable levels.

In order to deal more effectively with the discomfort of deprivation and the urge to smoke (i.e. without turning to food), Glenda would have had to develop an HFT philosophy and then act in ways that were consistent with this philosophy.

If Glenda could have articulated her HFT belief at the time she would have said something like this:

> It is difficult for me to put up with the discomfort of not having a cigarette when I want one, but I can put up with it and it is worth it to me to do so because not smoking is good for my health. Also, while I don't have to act on my urge to have a cigarette when I feel like having one, I also do not have to get rid of the urge. The urge will diminish if I do not act on it, although I realize that it will initially increase if I do not satisfy it. I also do not have to eat chocolate if I don't have a cigarette. If I do so, it will create another problem even if I do give up smoking. If I don't eat chocolate, I realize that my discomfort and the urge to rid myself of this discomfort will initially increase in strength. However, I also realize that after a while it will diminish if I tolerate it and just get on with the business of living.

Alternative healthy behaviours and the power of getting on with things

In this section, I want to consider (1) what makes an alternative behaviour healthy and (2) the power of getting on with things.

Alternative healthy behaviour

When you refrain from acting in a self-undisciplined way, it may help you to act in a healthy manner instead. As I have stressed, it is important that you first deal productively with the discomfort and the associated urge of not acting in a self-undisciplined way, and this is best done by rehearsing helpful HFT beliefs. After you do this, by all means act in an alternative way as long as it is healthy for you to do so. As I showed above, swapping one self-undisciplined behaviour for another is not the long-term answer to developing self-discipline. So what constitutes healthy alternative behaviour? I would say that it is healthy for you to engage in alternative behaviour if that behaviour satisfies the following criteria:

- It does not have unhealthy consequences for you.
- It perhaps helps you to achieve self-discipline in another area of your life.
- It is consistent with your values, if relevant.
- It promotes self-reliance.
- It does not reinforce your philosophy of LFT by distracting you from tolerating discomfort, for example.

The power of getting on with things

A different approach to addressing the issue of what to do after you have refrained from engaging in self-undisciplined behaviour can be summed up in the phrase: 'nothing special'. You just get on with the things that you are doing. You do not do anything that you would ordinarily not do in the situation in question.

For example, I discussed above the example of Glenda, who was trying to refrain from smoking. Ensuring that she did so for healthy reasons, Glenda decided that she would phone a friend for support and encouragement. This represented something specific that she could do instead of taking and smoking a cigarette, but it was something that she would not normally have done in the situation she was in. What I am suggesting here is that rather than doing something specific instead of taking a cigarette, Glenda just gets on with the business of interacting with the people she is with in the situation. Thus, she may continue to talk, drink (as long as this is not a distraction from dealing with the urge to smoke) and do all the things that she would normally do, without smoking a cigarette! This is particularly important for those like Glenda who associate self-undisciplined behaviour (like smoking) with other enjoyable activities that are not in themselves examples of self-undisciplined behaviour (e.g. laughing with friends, talking with friends, telling jokes or buying a round of drinks).

When she thought carefully about this issue, Glenda saw that she had unwittingly taught herself that she could not enjoy herself (e.g. laughing with friends, talking with smoking friends, telling jokes or buying a round of drinks) if she was not smoking a cigarette.

If she treats this as a fact then she will continue to smoke and thus trap herself in a self-fulfilling prophecy. However, if she regards it as a hypothesis, she will then resolve to carry out the four above-mentioned behaviours without smoking in order to see what happens. Glenda decided that she would do this experiment and found that although she felt awkward she could laugh and talk with her smoking friends, etc., without smoking herself. When she continued to practise enjoying herself without smoking, she also found that her sense of awkwardness diminished and disappeared after a while.

Do your own experiment

In order to carry out your own experiment in this area, I suggest that you do the following:

- Specify the desired behaviours that you think you cannot do without carrying out the self-undisciplined behaviour in question.
- Make sure that you only focus on desired behaviours that are not unhealthy for you.

- Resolve to carry out and actually execute the desired behaviours without engaging in the self-undisciplined behaviour that you wish to refrain from doing. Expect to feel awkward and uncomfortable when doing so.
- Did you do this? If not, how did you stop yourself from doing it? Deal with these obstacles and re-do the experiment.
- Continue in this vein until you have properly tested your hypothesis about carrying out the desired behaviour without engaging in the target self-undisciplined behaviour. You should conclude that you *can* carry out the desired behaviours without acting with self-indiscipline.
- Keep breaking the association between the desired behaviours and the target self-undisciplined behaviour until you are quite comfortable in carrying out the desired behaviours in the absence of the target self-undisciplined behaviour.

Perhaps the most important key to refraining from acting in self-undisciplined ways is to deal effectively with urges to act in these ways. This is the subject of the next chapter.

9

Deal with urges to engage in self-undisciplined behaviour

One of the most important skills that you can learn in your quest to develop self-discipline is to deal effectively with the urges that you experience to act in a self-undisciplined manner. These urges, of course, emanate from the short-term self (STS). If you act on these urges, doing so serves as a major obstacle to you as you work towards greater self-discipline.

Distinguish between urges and actions

One of the most important distinctions that you can make as you work towards becoming more self-disciplined is that between experiencing an urge to act in a self-undisciplined way and actually acting on that urge.

For example, I love chocolate, but I also want to keep my weight down. So, when I am at a party and someone brings round a box of chocolates and asks me if I want a chocolate, I have an urge to take one, but I do not act on that urge. Some people think that if they experience an urge to do something then they have to act on that urge. They literally do not distinguish between an urge to act and an overt action. This is what psychologists call the 'urge–act' fusion. In the minds of people who fuse an urge with an act, if they are to be self-disciplined then they have to eliminate their urges.

Unfortunately, attempts to eradicate urges are usually doomed to fail for two main reasons. First, such attempts are based on self-deception. To eliminate an urge, you have to persuade yourself that you don't want what you have an urge to have. Thus, when I experience an urge to take a chocolate when offered one, in order to eliminate this urge I would have to somehow persuade myself that I do not want a chocolate. This is a lie. I do want one. So this won't work in the long term.

The second reason that attempts to eliminate urges fail is that such attempts often have the opposite effect. Thus, if I try to eliminate my urge for chocolate, I may make the chocolate something forbidden and this makes it more attractive to me, not less.

Identify the form your urges take

An urge can be defined as a strong feeling that you experience to act in a certain way. However, people experience urges in different ways. For some, urges are physical sensations, while for others thoughts are major components of urges. Some experience images that accompany urges and see a sumptuous piece of cake in their mind's eye, while others do not have such mental pictures. It may be that your urges for different things come in different forms. However, if you focus on refraining from engaging in one self-undisciplined behaviour at a time, you will be able to identify the key components of your urge in that particular domain.

In general, urges can have the following components:

- *Feeling components*: these can be pleasant (in anticipation of engaging in the self-undisciplined behaviour) or unpleasant (if you don't act on your urge).
- *Sensation components*: again, these can be pleasant (in anticipation of engaging in the self-undisciplined behaviour) or unpleasant (if you don't act on your urge).
- *Thinking components*: these thoughts are either (a) rationalizations which seemingly provide 'good' reasons for self-undisciplined behaviour or (b) negative predictions of what will happen if you don't engage in this behaviour.
- *Imagery components*: these are mental pictures in which you see either (a) the positive features of engaging in self-undisciplined behaviour or (b) the negative features of not so engaging.
- *Behavioural components*: these occur in the form of (a) tendencies to act which you can either convert into overt action or not and (b) negative behaviour that you will engage in if you don't act on your urges.

Glenda's example
Glenda identified the following components of her urge to smoke when she refrained from accepting a cigarette in the bar, as discussed earlier:
1 *a physical component*: craving located in her mouth
2 *an imagery component*: an image of herself feeling a part of the social group and enjoying herself while smoking
3 *a behavioural component*: restless hands if she doesn't smoke.

Ten steps in dealing productively with urges

At the beginning of this chapter, I argued that trying to eliminate urges is generally counterproductive. As such, what is a more effective way of dealing with them? First, it is important that you build up a picture of when you experience urges to act in self-undisciplined ways. This involves monitoring your urges and linking them to situations you are in. This will enable you to anticipate when you are likely to experience these urges. Then you are ready to deal with these urges in productive ways. I suggest that you use the following steps in dealing with your urges.

Step 1: Acknowledge that you are experiencing an urge

Here it is important to draw upon the material I have just discussed and realize that you may experience an urge as a feeling, a sensation, a thought, an image and/or an impulse to act. Thus, when I am offered a chocolate, I experience a positive sensation (salivation) and an urge to take one (impulse to act). I acknowledge to myself that I do have this urge. I do not try to lie to myself, push the urge away or distract myself from the urge. Your urge is likely to be based on a desire to immediately experience a positive state (like the taste of chocolate) or to immediately eliminate a negative state (like anxiety which can be eliminated by inhaling cigarette smoke).

Step 2: Acknowledge that the urge is difficult to tolerate, but that you can tolerate it and that it is worth tolerating

The urge I experience when I am offered a chocolate is tolerable. This is a fact independent of whether I believe it or not, and it is worth it to me to tolerate it because doing so will help me to maintain my weight.

Believing that you can tolerate urges and that it is worth it to you to do so is known as a high frustration tolerance (HFT) belief. In general, an HFT belief is true since this is made up of the following ideas:

- I will struggle if the frustration or discomfort continues to exist, but I will neither die nor disintegrate.
- I will not lose the capacity to experience happiness if the frustration or discomfort continues to exist, although this capacity will be temporarily diminished.
- The frustration or discomfort is worth tolerating. (Here, you need to specify in which ways this is the case.)

Step 3: Acknowledge that you do not have to act on your urge immediately

One of the reasons you have developed self-indiscipline in a given area is that your behaviour in this area has been based on the idea that you have to act on your urge immediately. The good news is that you don't have to do so. You are not a slave to your urges. It is possible for you to experience an urge and not immediately act on it. If you refrain from acting on your urge, you will find that the urge will initially increase in intensity but later decrease if you continue to refrain from acting on it. Taking the previous step will help you to do that.

Step 4: Recognize that you have a choice: to act on the urge or not

Once you have given yourself some breathing space by refraining from acting on the urge as soon as you experience it, you then can stand back and use your urge as a cue to recognize that you have a choice. You can act on the urge or not.

Step 5: Remind yourself of the positive reasons for refraining from acting on such urges and the negative reasons for acting on them

Having recognized that you can choose to act on the urge or not, engage your executive self (ES) and review the reasons why it is in your best interests not to act on it. Remind yourself of the benefits of such restraint and the costs of urge-based action (see Chapter 4).

Step 6: Respond to any positive reasons for acting on your urge and to any negative reasons against refraining from doing so

It may be that while you are deciding whether or not to act on your urge, your STS provides you with reasons to act on the urge. When this happens, it is useful to respond to them whether they are positive reasons for acting on the urge or negative reasons against refraining from doing so. If your STS becomes fully activated and keeps attacking healthy responses, it is important that you acknowledge the existence of these STS-based counter-arguments and then proceed to the next step.

Step 7: Take purposive action even though you are experiencing the urge

As I pointed out above, refraining from acting on your urge eventually leads to a decrease in that urge's intensity. This process is hastened if you take purposive action even though you are experiencing the urge. If you believe that you cannot take such action until you have eliminated the urge, then fortunately you are wrong. It is quite possible for you to take purposive action even though you are experiencing an urge. Thus, I can converse with a person at a party even though I have an urge to eat chocolate. Indeed, once you engage in purposive action, you are increasingly able to focus your attention on this activity once you have accepted the existence of the urge and that you don't have to satisfy it or get rid of it.

So what I am talking about here is not distraction from the urge.

That would involve you trying to get rid of it. Rather, I am talking about a process of moving forward with the urge, while doing nothing about it. You neither act to satisfy it, nor distract yourself from it. You just let it be. Yes, it is more difficult than it sounds, but it is worthwhile cultivating this habit.

Step 8: Ask yourself, 'Did I act on the urge or not?'

This calls for a straightforward 'yes' or 'no' answer. However, it is important for you to realize that you may have compensated for successfully refraining from acting on the urge in the situation under investigation. For example, you may have refrained from acting on the urge to smoke, but compensated for it by drinking too much. If this is the case, and you do this routinely, you may benefit from professional help since this level of complexity is beyond the scope of this book.

Step 9: Ask yourself, 'If I acted on the urge, what were my true reasons for doing so?'

If you acted on your urge in an area where it would have been in your healthy interests not to do so, it is important for you to be honest with yourself and identify the true reasons (as far as you are aware of them) for doing so. I have worked with people with self-discipline problems for over 30 years, and one of the 'givens' about working with this group of people is their capacity for self-deception and rationalization. I will deal with this more extensively later in this chapter, but for now I will note that if you acted on your urge you may well try to deceive yourself and others by coming up with what you think is a good reason why you acted on the urge, but what is in fact a rationalization.

The difference between a good reason and a rationalization is this:

A *good reason* for acting on your urge is one that is true and reasonable as judged by a jury of objective observers in possession of all the facts (e.g. 'I acted on my urge because if I had not done so my children would have been severely penalized' – where this was found to be accurate).

A *rationalization* for acting on your urge is one that is unreasonable as judged by a jury of objective observers in possession of all the facts (e.g. 'I acted on my urge because I thought I deserved a treat').

Step 10: Rate immediate and later changes in the intensity of the urge (on a scale from 1 to 10)

As you work towards developing greater self-discipline, you need to understand two important points:

- If you act on your urge you will rid yourself of the urge and thus reduce its intensity, but this is at a great price – you do not develop self-discipline, which is largely based on not acting on urges to behave in self-defeating ways.
- If you refrain from acting on your urge, the intensity of this urge will temporarily increase, but if you involve yourself in productive action while experiencing the urge without acting on it, then the intensity of the urge will decrease.

I suggest that you test the truth or falsity of these points by using a 1–10 scale to rate the intensity of an urge at two stages: (1) immediately after you have decided not to act on the urge and (2) at a later stage.

I have developed a form, a blank version of which can be found in Appendix 6, which can be used in situations in which you are experiencing an urge or as an 'after the event' analysis of how you dealt with it. I will now show the way Glenda and Colin used the form in detailing how they responded to urges to smoke a cigarette and to avoid working on an essay, respectively.

Dealing with urges: Glenda's example
We met Glenda earlier. She wanted to give up smoking. Here is how she used the above ten principles to deal with her urges to smoke.

Date: *6/5/06* Time: *6.05 p.m.*
Situation: *I was in the wine bar across the street from work. I had just begun to unwind with a glass of red wine when someone offered me a cigarette*
Alone/with others: *With my smoking friends from work*
Nature of the urge: *To smoke a cigarette*
Strength of urge (1–10): *7*
Purpose of the urge: *To unwind even more*

1 Acknowledge that you are experiencing an urge.
   I acknowledged that I was experiencing a strongish urge, which I felt in my throat, to smoke a cigarette.

2 Acknowledge that the urge is difficult to tolerate, but that you can tolerate it and that it is worth tolerating.
   I told myself that I can tolerate this urge and that I don't have to get rid of it immediately. I also told myself it was in my interests to tolerate the urge in that it will help me to achieve my goals.

3 Acknowledge that you do not have to act on your urge immediately.
   I told my friend that I wouldn't have one there and then, but that I might have one later.

4 Recognize that you have a choice: to act on the urge or not.
   *Telling my friend that I would not have one at that moment helped me
   in two ways. It gave me time to think, and by refusing I saw that I didn't
   have to have a cigarette whenever I drink red wine in the company of
   my smoking friends.*

5 Remind yourself of the positive reasons for refraining from acting on
   such urges and the negative reasons for acting on them.
   *I reminded myself that I didn't want to drink much that evening and
   I drink less when I don't smoke. I also reminded myself that I want to
   improve my health.*

6 Respond to any positive reasons for acting on your urge and to any
   negative reasons against refraining from doing so.
   *I recognized that smoking in these circumstances may make me appear
   cool, but this is a transitory effect and is not worth doing since probably
   it is only me that thinks that I am cool – and that is only an illusion
   anyway. I also reminded myself that smoking is not the only reason for
   our collective friendship and therefore I don't have to smoke to feel part
   of the group. We are friends because we like each other's company and
   we enjoy stimulating conversation. If we all smoked but the last two
   factors were absent, then we would not be friends.*

7 Take purposive action even though you are experiencing the urge.
   *I kept my mind on the great conversation that we were having even
   though I was aware of the urge at the back of my mind.*

8 Ask yourself, 'Did I act on the urge or not?'
   I did not smoke the cigarette when it was offered.

9 Ask yourself, 'If I acted on the urge, what were my true reasons for
   doing so?'
   Not relevant.

10 Rate the immediate and later changes in the intensity of the urge
    (1–10).
    *Once I refrained from acting on the urge it went up to 8; after 15
    minutes it had come down to 2.*

Comments

Glenda's report of how to refrain from acting on an urge is excellent and can be used as a model of this skill. Note how Glenda was able to put into practice all the relevant skills that I discussed above. In particular, it is worthwhile noting that the intensity of Glenda's urge increased from 7 to 8 as she initially refrained from acting on her urge, but then decreased markedly from 8 to 2 as she continued to do so.

Dealing with urges: Colin's example

Date: *16/6/06* Time: *7.03 p.m.*
Situation: *I was at home in my study having committed myself to doing the essay I had been putting off*
Alone/with others: *Alone*
Nature of the urge: *To tidy my desk before getting down to work*
Strength of urge (1–10): *6*
Purpose of the urge: *To avoid the discomfort of getting down to work*

1 Acknowledge that you are experiencing an urge.
I acknowledged that I was experiencing a strong behavioural urge to get away from doing my work by tidying my desk.

2 Acknowledge that the urge is difficult to tolerate, but that you can tolerate it and that it is worth tolerating.
I tried to tell myself that I can put up with this urge, but I didn't really believe it. I didn't try to convince myself that it was worth it to tolerate the urge.

3 Acknowledge that you do not have to act on your urge immediately.
I stopped myself from tidying before picking up my pencil in order to sharpen it. In doing so, I saw that I did not have to engage in tidying.

4 Recognize that you have a choice: to act on the urge or not.
I reminded myself that I had a choice to get down to the work or put it off by tidying my desk.

5 Remind yourself of the positive reasons for refraining from acting on such urges and the negative reasons for acting on them.
I reminded myself that in this context tidying up is not work. It is intended to be a way of delaying work which has to be done anyway, so I might as well do it sooner than later.

6 Respond to any positive reasons for acting on your urge and to any negative reasons against refraining from doing so.
I did not do this because at this point I was beginning to feel rebellious (see below).

7 Take purposive action even though you are experiencing the urge.
The idea was that I would work even though I wanted to delay it. However, I did not do it.

8 Ask yourself, 'Did I act on the urge or not?'
I did act on the urge to tidy my room and, once again, I did not get around to working on my essay. I persuaded myself that I needed to tidy my room in order to concentrate on writing my essay.

9 Ask yourself, 'If I acted on the urge, what were my true reasons for doing so?'
I felt rebellious, so I guess I was trying to show myself that I had the freedom to do what I wanted to do.

10 Rate the immediate and later changes in the intensity of the urge (1–10).
By acting on the urge, I satisfied it and it disappeared.

Comments

Colin failed on this occasion to refrain from acting on the urge to tidy his study rather than work on his essay. If we look carefully at Colin's form, the reasons he acted on his urge to avoid working on his essay by tidying his study are clear. The first point where Colin's attempt to deal constructively with his urge to avoid starting work on his essay broke down was when he tried to tell himself that he could tolerate this urge, but that he didn't really believe this. In order to accept this high frustration tolerance (HFT) belief, Colin would have had to convince himself that this belief was true, sensible and helpful, and act in ways that were consistent with it. Then later he started to feel rebellious. His rebelliousness and his decision to act on it was, as Colin notes, a way of helping him gain a sense that he was free to act as he pleased. This highlights the fact that Colin has to learn to deal constructively with his urge to act on his rebellious feelings if he is to develop greater self-discipline.

Pseudo work as rationalization

Colin rationalizes tidying his desk by persuading himself that such behaviour is a part of his work rather than an avoidance of it. His tidying is thus an example of pseudo work, which is behaviour that appears to be a part of the self-disciplined task. It is, in Colin's case and often more generally, an example of procrastination. Pseudo work is therefore an act of self-deception which can also be used to deceive others and is often backed up by related rationalizations (e.g. 'I couldn't concentrate on my essay when my study was so untidy, so I tidied my study first').

How can you tell if an activity is work (an intrinsic part of the task associated with self-discipline) or pseudo work (a task that is connected to the task but which serves, in reality, as a way of avoiding it)? Here are a few guidelines, and I will refer to Colin's example to illustrate my points.

- Can you engage in the main task without first engaging in the task that you actually carried out?
  Colin's example: Can Colin work on his essay without first tidying his study? The answer here is 'yes', and thus tidying his study is pseudo work and is therefore an avoidant activity.

- Would an independent jury in possession of all the facts say that the task that you engaged in was work or pseudo work?
  Colin's example: In the case of Colin and with the evidence available to them (including (a) his stated goals, (b) the fact that tidying his room was not, on this occasion, a prelude to work but an avoidance of it and (c) his dealing with urges form – see pp. 99–100), a jury would in all probability conclude that tidying his room was an example of pseudo work and not work.

- Was the task that you engaged in an expression of an urge that is usually associated with self-indiscipline?
  Colin's example: Is tidying his room something that Colin routinely does as a prelude to work, or does he generally use this as a way of avoiding getting down to work? In this case, Colin admitted to himself that tidying his study is generally associated with, and an expression of, an urge to avoid doing his work.

Dealing productively with urges is *not* a one-off event

Once you have dealt with an urge using the above steps in one given situation, you will still have to deal with urges in the same or similar situations. Humans routinely have urges to act in self-undisciplined ways, and the best response to this fact is not to eliminate such urges from the human experience – a task that would be impossible – but to accept this as grim reality and learn to deal with urges on an ongoing basis.

Once you have successfully applied the above steps a number of times when you experience urges to act in self-undisciplined ways, you can then improvise with the steps and choose those that are particularly effective for you. Your goal should be to use those steps that are personally effective and that can be quickly applied in situations when you experience urges.

Acting on an urge as an unproductive coping strategy

There is one phenomenon that I particularly wish to bring to your attention and discuss with respect to dealing with urges. I do so because it is something that I encounter a lot in my practice with clients who ask me to help them develop greater self-discipline. These clients say that they act on their urges because if they don't do so they will then obsess about the object of their urges.

For example, Simon was working towards developing healthier eating patterns, but he often experienced urges to eat high fat, high cholesterol food. Although Simon followed the steps outlined above, he still acted on his urges and ate these foods which were against his self-disciplined objectives. When Simon reflected on this experience, he realized that he ate these foods in order to stop himself from obsessing about them later. I helped Simon to realize that he was holding a rigid belief about his food preferences that led him to obsess about these foods. He expressed this belief as 'I must have the food that I want, and I can't stand being deprived.' Simon learned, therefore, that it was not being deprived of his desired food that led him to obsess, but his rigid belief about this deprivation. As a result, I helped Simon to target this rigid belief for change, and when he did this he realized that he could deprive himself of his desired food without obsessing about it.

Self-reward and self-blame

When you have experienced an urge and refrained from acting on it, you need to congratulate yourself for succeeding at something you have previously failed at. It is very easy to overlook doing so. Human beings find it much easier to blame themselves when they make mistakes than to congratulate themselves for acting well. You may think that you are being weak or childish for congratulating yourself. If so, think again. If you were managing a team at work, would you get more from them by praising them for their good performance or blaming them for their bad performance? There are many psychology studies to show that praise is better than blame for getting the most out of people. However, just because you praised your team when they were doing well, it does not follow that you would ignore their errors. No! You would bring these errors to their attention and help them to learn from them. The fact that you would be doing so from the basis of praise for good performance would mean that you would increase the chances that your team members would listen to your feedback, designed as it is to help them to correct their errors.

The same goes with acquiring self-discipline: if you only blame yourself when you act on your urges and never praise yourself for times when you have refrained from acting on these urges, then you will easily get discouraged. With such feelings of discouragement, you are more likely to act in self-undisciplined ways in order to cheer yourself up. Thus, self-blame often leads to greater self-indiscipline.

My advice therefore is to praise yourself whenever you refrain from acting on your self-undisciplined urges, and accept yourself but take responsibility for when you do act on them. This attitude will help you to focus on the specific episode of self-indiscipline and learn from your experiences of self-discipline failure. The trouble with blaming yourself for acting on your urges is that you become so preoccupied with how lazy, weak or uncontrolled you are that you have little remaining mental space to learn from your experiences.

Use imagery practice in dealing with urges

In Chapter 5, I discussed how to use imagery methods to help you rehearse acting in self-disciplined ways. You can also use these imagery methods to practise dealing productively with urges. You might like to review this material now if you need to.

Let me demonstrate the use of imagery in dealing with urges by showing how I use it in my own life.

1 *Anticipate the situation in which the urge is likely to be experienced.*
Tomorrow evening I am going out to dinner with my wife and another couple and I anticipate that a plate of delicious bread will be served with the hors d'oeuvres.
2 *Locate the urge.*
I anticipate experiencing the urge in my mouth and behaviourally, with my hand reaching to take a slice of bread.
3 *Picture yourself rehearsing healthy attitudes with respect to the urge and refraining from the self-undisciplined action.*
I see myself telling myself: 'I want the bread, but I don't need it and I am going to choose not to have it.' I also picture myself telling myself: 'I can stand the urge and I don't have to do anything to get rid of it,' as the strength of the urge temporarily increases as a result of me not taking the bread.

4 *Review the reasons for refraining from acting in self-undisciplined ways, if necessary.*
   I did not have to do this.
5 *Reward yourself in some way.*
   I picture myself being pleased that I have acted in self-disciplined ways and have not eaten the bread, telling myself: 'Well done, Windy, you acted in a self-disciplined manner.'

In the next chapter, I will discuss three important issues concerning how you can best implement a self-discipline programme based on refraining from acting in self-undisciplined ways.

10

Refrain from acting in a self-undisciplined manner

In this chapter, I will discuss three issues that are relevant to how you can approach the business of refraining from engaging in activities in a self-undisciplined manner. First, I will discuss whether you should refrain from acting in a self-undisciplined way immediately and fully (colloquially known as 'going cold turkey') or whether you should cut down gradually until you have reached your self-discipline goal. Second, I will discuss what you can do if you just can't keep to your self-discipline goal. Finally, I will discuss what you can do if you want to refrain from acting in a self-undisciplined manner in several areas: should you change one thing at a time or should you target for change all the areas at once?

'Going cold turkey' vs. cutting down gradually until you reach your goal

When you set a self-discipline goal that relates to refraining from acting in a self-undisciplined manner, you need to decide how you are going to achieve your goal. There are basically two choices here: give up completely and immediately ('going cold turkey') or cut down until you have reached your goal. In the literature on self-discipline you will find advocates of both positions. My own view is that it is important that you understand the advantages and disadvantages of both approaches before deciding on which approach best suits you and has the greatest chance of success from a long-term perspective.

'Going cold turkey'

As I have stated, 'going cold turkey' means that when you have decided to refrain from acting in a self-undisciplined manner, you do so immediately and completely. This is the approach advocated by Alcoholics Anonymous (AA). They argue that as alcoholism is an illness, it makes no sense to attempt to cut down on a substance that is making you ill. Better therefore to aim to 'go cold turkey' and get intensive support from AA in the process. It is my view that the reason AA is effective for some people is that it offers an intensive level of support. Thus, members of AA can go to daily meetings and can phone a 'sponsor' (i.e. a person who mentors them through the recovery process) when they feel vulnerable to using alcohol. So let me first discuss the advantages of the 'cold turkey' approach to refraining from acting in a self-undisciplined manner.

Advantages of 'going cold turkey'

'Going cold turkey' is an ambitious approach to developing self-discipline based on refraining from acting in a self-undisciplined manner. It has a number of advantages.

It offers a quick route to self-discipline By definition, when you 'go cold turkey', you can reach your self-discipline goal immediately. Thus, if you want to achieve your goal very quickly and you think that you can do this, then 'going cold turkey' may be for you. Be aware, though, that there is a greater chance of failure with this approach than with a more gradual approach to self-discipline where you refrain from acting in a self-undisciplined manner.

However, if you experience early success with a 'cold turkey' approach to refraining-based self-discipline, you are likely to feel greatly encouraged by your success and this encouragement may serve as a powerful motivator for the longer haul.

When intensive support is offered you have a better chance of success If you are going to 'go cold turkey' then you will increase your chances of success if you have others to support you in your self-disciplined endeavours. I mentioned above that one of the reasons AA is effective (when it is so) is the intensive level of support offered to those who in effect 'go cold turkey' in abstaining completely from alcohol. When you 'go cold turkey', you need support, for a number of reasons. First, the intensity of the urge to act in a self-undisciplined manner is likely to be greater with a 'cold turkey' regime than with a more gradual approach to giving up, and therefore having someone to whom you can turn for support in dealing with these urges is useful. For example, in AA, each member has a sponsor to whom he or she can turn in times of vulnerability. Dealing with urges to engage in self-undisciplined behaviour is perhaps the Achilles' heel of most people who have set a self-discipline goal, and particularly so when you are 'going cold turkey'. Choosing a person who you think will be supportive is an important issue and one that I will consider in greater depth in the next chapter. In AA, the advantage of having a sponsor for support is that this person will know what you are going through. He or she will be a 'recovering alcoholic' and will have experienced wrestling with urges to drink (in this case). A sponsor, therefore, provides an informed level of support, and it is this knowledge gained through experience that AA members often refer to when discussing the help a sponsor provides.

So, if you are 'going cold turkey', set up a support network for yourself. Choose someone or a group of people genuinely on your side and supportive of your self-discipline goals and, preferably, knowledgeable of the problems that you are likely to encounter by 'going cold turkey', and who can thus offer you informed support.

Disadvantages of 'going cold turkey'

While 'going cold turkey' can help you to achieve your self-discipline goals quite quickly, it does have a number of disadvantages.

It tends to have a high level of failure   This book is based on the idea that you enhance the chances of developing self-discipline when you acquire and practise a number of healthy attitudes and behavioural skills, which I discuss throughout. When you 'go cold turkey' you need to use these skills straight away, particularly to deal productively with the urges that you will, in all probability, experience. The trouble is that if you 'go cold turkey', you will not have had the chance to embed these attitudes and skills in your response repertoire sufficiently to use them straight away. If you do not use these skills then you will increase the chances that you will 'fall back' and act in a self-undisciplined manner.

You rely heavily on environmental control   Thus, when you 'go cold turkey' you are not yet sufficiently well equipped to use the attitudes and skills needed to develop self-discipline. As such, if you are to remain on this regime then you will become increasingly reliant on controlling your environment as a way of developing self-discipline. Unable to make use of self-disciplined beliefs and skills, your best bet is to avoid the temptation of acting in a self-undisciplined manner. This means avoiding environments where you previously engaged in the target behaviour. Thus, if you were abstaining immediately from alcohol, you would avoid places where alcohol is served and can be purchased, and the same with high calorie food. If you were 'going cold turkey' with gambling, you would avoid going to casinos, bookmakers', dog tracks and racecourses. You would avoid logging on to internet gambling sites and even avoid going into places that sell lottery tickets. And if you were refraining immediately from smoking you would avoid shops that sell cigarettes and avoid places where smoking is permitted. On this latter point, the legislation which came into force on 1 July 2007 in England (and a little earlier in Scotland and Wales), where smoking is not permitted in indoor public places, has undoubtedly helped many people who hitherto smoked to give up.

The problem with developing self-discipline based on environmental control is twofold. First, you cannot perfectly control your environment. Thus, you may be at an indoor event where smoking is prohibited, but meet friends you have not seen for a long time, some of whom smoke, and they invite you to go out for a chat and a smoke. Or you may avoid obvious places where gambling takes place, but then be offered raffle tickets at a church social. If you have not developed the attitudes and skills underpinning self-discipline, then you may well engage in these behaviours when it is not wise for you to do so if environmental control lets you down.

Second, you may wittingly or unwittingly place yourself in environments where you will experience temptation to engage in behaviours that may lead to self-indiscipline. For example, Jeremy had targeted refraining from drinking alcohol as his self-discipline goal. He was successful at staying away from pubs and wine bars, but chose to attend a book launch where he knew, if he was honest with himself, that alcohol would be served. As a consequence, he ended up by getting drunk. When discussing this episode at a local AA meeting, he claimed at first that he had not known that alcohol would be served at the book launch. However, he was confronted on this by some of the other AA members and admitted that (1) alcohol had been served at every book launch he had ever attended and (2) he had planned on going and drinking 'just the one glass of wine'. This is a good example of how it is easy for you to deceive yourself as you struggle to develop refraining-based self-discipline. You need to be completely honest with yourself if you are to maximize the chances of achieving these self-discipline goals.

You rely on external means of developing self-discipline When you choose to 'go cold turkey' and have not developed any self-discipline skills, you will tend to rely on external means of developing self-discipline. Examples of such means include the following:

- using nicotine patches and Zyban (a prescription drug) to help you refrain from smoking;
- using Antabuse (a prescription drug that induces vomiting if you drink) to help you refrain from drinking alcohol;
- taking spirulina tablets to develop a full feeling in your stomach so that you do not eat to excess;

- having your stomach stapled to help you refrain from eating excessively;
- going out with no money or credit cards so that you cannot gamble or shop.

While some of these external methods of developing self-discipline may be necessary (e.g. stomach stapling when everything else has failed and your health or life is significantly at risk), most of them are fraught with problems. Thus, you may easily stop using patches and go back to smoking, or you may borrow money so that you can gamble or shop, when you are in certain environments where you think that you cannot or do not want to 'resist' the urge to act in a self-undisciplined manner.

Also, when you use these methods you are unwittingly reinforcing the idea that you are weak and cannot learn to develop self-discipline without the use of such external methods.

Cutting down gradually until you reach your goal

The main alternative to 'going cold turkey' in the development of refraining-based self-discipline is the 'cutting down gradually until you reach your goal' approach. This goal may mean completely refraining from an activity (e.g. abstaining from drinking alcohol) or it may involve you allowing yourself to engage occasionally in the activity (e.g. drinking three glasses of wine a week). As with the 'going cold turkey' approach, the gradual approach has advantages and disadvantages.

Advantages of cutting down gradually until you reach your goal

The gradual approach to developing self-discipline based on refraining from acting in a self-undisciplined manner has a number of advantages.

It is rooted in realism

As I discussed above, 'going cold turkey' is very demanding and most people fail to refrain from acting in a self-undisciplined manner by taking this approach. As Mark Twain said: 'Giving up smoking is easy, I've done it hundreds of times.' By contrast, the gradual approach to refraining-based self-discipline is less demanding and therefore more realistic, and more people are likely to succeed in the longer term in using it. This is not to say that it does not have its problems, for it does, as I will discuss below. But it does not expect you to go from self-indiscipline to self-discipline in one jump, and as such it acknowledges that self-discipline is something that needs to be practised and developed gradually rather than attempted 'in one go'.

It allows for the gradual practice of the beliefs and skills of self-discipline

As I have just stated in the previous point, the gradual approach allows you to develop self-discipline gradually. More importantly, it allows you to practise the beliefs and skills that I have discussed in this book, and to practise them under increasingly difficult circumstances. Thus, if you have as your self-discipline goal refraining from drinking more than one glass of wine a day, you might start by reducing your daily wine intake from your starting position (say, five glasses) to four glasses and planning on where and when you will consume these glasses. Then you will practise dealing productively with your urges at other times, in the way that I discussed in Chapter 9. When you feel more competent at using these skills, you might use them when you have reduced your intake to three glasses a day, and continue in this vein until you have achieved your goal.

It is easier to learn from lapses

If you are working towards a refraining-based self-discipline goal using either a 'cold turkey' approach or a gradual approach, the reality is that you will at some point lapse. I define a lapse as a momentary return to self-undisciplined behaviour, while a relapse is a more enduring and significant 'back to square one' return to self-undisciplined behaviour. If you are undertaking a gradual approach to refraining-based self-discipline then it is easier to learn from your lapses, because you can pinpoint more keenly what was going on when you lapsed. As your progress is more gradual, you can more easily understand why you returned momentarily to self-undisciplined behaviour than if you have 'gone cold turkey'. The latter is an either–or approach, and the reasons for lapsing are therefore more numerous and harder to identify.

Disadvantages of cutting down gradually until you stop
You are still engaging with self-undisciplined activities

One of the biggest drawbacks to a gradual approach to achieving a refraining-based self-discipline goal is that as you work towards this goal you are still engaging in self-undisciplined behaviour, albeit with reducing frequency. As such, you are still practising the very behaviour you are striving to refrain from. For some, this is problematic, and if this applies to you, you may be suited to a 'cold turkey' approach. For others, the gradual approach is a comfort, because they gain confidence as they gradually cut down on their way to their goals.

It can be harder to see the line between control and lack of control

One of my clients – let me call him Eric – wanted to be able to 'drink sensibly' as his self-discipline goal, by which he meant three units of alcohol per day. The trouble was that when he had had two units, his ability to see the difference between what he considered to be control (i.e. three units) and lack of control (in his view more than three units) was diminished. His experience taught him that he had to revise his goal. He decided to have just one drink because he learned that when he had two, he was quite likely to drink more! While Eric had the flexibility to revise his self-discipline goal, many people who want to continue engaging in behaviour (e.g. drinking and smoking) that is problematic for them when done excessively lack this flexibility. Consequently, the gradual approach to achieving refraining-based self-discipline goals may only serve to encourage them to maintain their self-undisciplined behaviour because they have chosen unrealistic goals they are unable to meet, Thus, if Eric was rigid about his goals and wanted to drink three units a day, his difficulty at thinking clearly having had two units would have served only to maintain his self-indiscipline.

You are more likely to engage in self-deception

Related to the above point, if you have set refraining-based goals that you can't achieve through adopting the gradual approach and you won't revise your goals, then you are very likely to engage in self-deception to justify your failures to achieve your unrealistic goals. Thus, if Eric had not revised his goals and kept trying, but failing, to stick to drinking three units of alcohol a day, then I could imagine that he might have said some of the following to explain his failures:

- 'It was a special occasion and I wanted to enjoy myself.'
- 'People were buying me drinks and it was rude to say "no".'
- 'I deserved to let my hair down after working so hard.'
- 'I lost count.'
- 'I forgot to remind myself what my goals were.'

Let me remind you that I am not advocating one approach over the other here. What I do suggest is that you are mindful of the advantages and disadvantages of both approaches, particularly as they apply to your unique situation. If in doubt, experiment with both and see which is more likely to help you achieve your self-discipline goals.

Abstinence vs. harm reduction

If you have set a self-discipline goal based on refraining from engaging in self-undisciplined behaviour, then you need to decide whether you are going to abstain from this activity or cut down on it while falling short of abstinence. The trouble with cutting down on a harmful activity is that it is still unhealthy, even if reduced, and for this reason many authorities in the self-discipline field recommend abstinence as a goal. However, some people for one reason or another either do not want to or are not capable (or think they are not capable) of achieving an abstinence goal, and therefore their only viable alternative is to go for a cutting-down goal or what is known in the literature as harm reduction.

As the term implies, harm reduction involves a compromise between abstinence and continuing to engage in a harmful activity. It involves continuing engagement but at a reduced level. Harm reduction was developed as an approach to help problem substance-abusers who had a very high rate of relapse in abstinence programmes, but it has latterly been used more widely in the general area of self-discipline.

For those able to achieve it, abstinence from engaging in self-undisciplined behaviour is the preferred option. Whether you achieve abstinence by 'going cold turkey' or by gradual cutting down until you have stopped, by abstaining from engaging in your target self-undisciplined behaviour you have achieved healthier goals than if you are working on a harm reduction programme. Thus, if you have stopped smoking you are protecting your lungs more than if you are still smoking, albeit at a reduced, less harmful rate. And if you have cut out very fatty foods, you are doing your arteries a bigger favour than if you have cut down on them. So then why wouldn't you go for abstinence? There are a number of reasons you might not.

Reasons people do not aim for abstinence

First, you may just not want to abstain from engaging in the self-undisciplined behaviour. Thus, you may enjoy smoking and want to continue to smoke even though you know it is harmful to you and to those around you. If this is the case, you might opt initially for a harm reduction programme (the main features of which are discussed below) and then review whether you want to opt for abstinence later.

Second, you may want to abstain but think that you won't be able to achieve it. If this is the case, you might start by opting for harm reduction. If you manage to reduce the harm you experience and reduce the extent to which you engage in self-undisciplined behaviour, then this may give you the confidence to switch to abstinence later.

Third, you may privately know that abstinence is the best option for you, but because you know that society at large values this, and perhaps because others want you to achieve it as well, to opt for an abstinence goal means to you that you are being controlled in some way. You thus rebel against this 'control' and refuse to opt for abstinence. If this is the case for you, it is important that you distinguish between reactance and independence. Reactance means that you rebel against something to assert your sense of freedom, even when this means doing things that you don't want to do and that are against your own judged best interests. Independence involves you acting in ways that are in your own judged best interests even when others force you to act in these ways. Here, you are asserting your sense of freedom by doing something that is right for you rather than going against the other. Interestingly, people who are highly reactant are quite easy to manipulate. Let's suppose that you are highly reactant and I want you to give up smoking. What I would do is to put pressure on you to smoke. In order for you to 'feel' that you were free, you would have to give up smoking – which is what I wanted you to do in the first place!

So, if you want to be independent in the field of self-discipline, do what you want to do irrespective of the views of and pressures from other people.

What harm reduction involves

As I mentioned earlier, when you are engaged on a harm reduction programme you seek to reduce the harm that you experience when you act in a self-undisciplined manner without fully giving up engaging in the behaviour. Thus, when you do engage in that behaviour you are looking to do so in ways that reduce that harm.

Take, for example, the case of Joanne. She often drank to excess, but rather than abstaining from alcohol, she opted to continue to drink but to reduce the harm she derived from drinking. In her case, this meant implementing the following strategies, which are intended to illustrate the harm reduction approach in action.

- When Joanne drank alone, she would limit herself to two glasses of wine and alternate one glass of wine with one glass of water. If she was tempted to drink a third glass she would practise her non-dogmatic preference and associated HFT belief thus: 'I would like a third glass of wine, but I don't have to have one. I can stand the deprivation of not meeting my desire.' If this failed she would phone a friend who would distract her from her urge to drink, or she would go for a walk round the block. If this failed and she drank a third glass she would have a spritzer (white wine mixed with soda water the same size as a glass of wine) rather than an undiluted glass of wine.

- When Joanne drank with others on a night out, she would limit herself to three glasses of wine for the evening. Before meeting her friends she would drink plenty of water, a strategy that she found useful in diminishing her desire for alcohol. If that did not work, she would alternate water and wine and make sure that she ate plenty of vegetable snacks rather than the available salty snacks. She would arrange for a taxi to pick her up before the others went on for a curry (which was always accompanied by more wine) and didn't accept or issue invitations to 'go back to mine', which again was the setting for more alcohol. If, as happened more than once, the taxi did not arrive and she went on for a curry she would order weak white wine spritzers (far more soda than wine) and if she went back to one of her friends' for a late night drink, she had a whisky, which she hated and invariably could only drink one mouthful.

I hope that Joanne's experiences have made clear the basic principle of harm reduction, which in a nutshell is this: if you can't or don't want to abstain from engaging in self-undisciplined behaviour, then at every opportunity reduce or minimize the harm you experience through engaging in that behaviour. And don't forget that at any time you can switch to an abstinence-based approach or experiment with one to see what happens, safe in the knowledge that you can always go back to harm reduction if abstinence fails or is not for you.

How many areas of self-indiscipline should you work on at any one time?

When you are setting self-discipline goals that involve you refraining from acting in self-undisciplined ways, it may be the case that, while you have only one area of self-indiscipline that you target for change, you have problems in more than one area of self-indiscipline. As such, you may wish to set more than one goal, and in some cases you may have several goals for change. If you have more than one goal in this respect, then you have to make a choice between working on one area of self-indiscipline at a time, working on more than one or indeed working on all of them at the same time.

For the last two years, Boots, the British retail chemist chain of stores, have run a campaign just after Christmas that targets people who want to set self-discipline goals as a New Year resolution. This campaign is called 'Change One Thing' and is based on the view that you are more likely to be successful at reaching one refraining-based self-discipline goal at a time than at reaching more than one goal or several such goals at a time. This is probably true for most people, but it is not true for all. So, if you have set more than one refraining-based self-discipline goal, how do you know if you should work on one at a time, more than one at a time or whether you should work on everything at once (what I call striving for self-discipline across the board)? The answer is that you do not know for sure at the outset which is the best approach for you to take. However, here are a number of points that you need to consider before making your decision. In considering these points, remember that you will be using the strategies and techniques that I have already outlined in this book. So if you have failed at previous attempts to work towards refraining-based goals, remember that this time will hopefully be different – you will be using methods derived from CBT which, in all probability, you have never used before.

1   Choose to work at one refraining-based self-discipline goal at a time if:
   (a) you have no prior experience at working towards a refraining-based self-discipline goal;
   (b) your previous attempts at working towards a single refraining-based self-discipline goal have never really got off the ground or have ended in failure quite quickly;
   (c) your confidence level at working towards one refraining-based self-discipline goal is low;
   (d) your confidence level at working towards a single refraining-based self-discipline goal is high, but you don't have confidence at tackling more than one problem behaviour at a time;
   (e) you find it difficult to apply general concepts to specific situations;
   (f) you prefer the idea of working on one refraining-based self-discipline goal at a time to working with more than one at a time or working towards self-discipline across the board.
2   Choose to work at more than one refraining-based self-discipline goal at a time if:
   (a) you have prior experience at working towards a refraining-based self-discipline goal and you have had some success in this area;
   (b) your confidence level at working towards more than one refraining-based self-discipline goal is quite high;
   (c) you can apply general concepts to specific situations;
   (d) you prefer the idea of working on more than one refraining-based self-discipline goal at a time to working on only one at a time, but you don't like the idea of working towards self-discipline across the board.
3   Choose to strive towards self-discipline across the board if:
   (a) you have a very good reason or set of reasons to do so;
   (b) you have prior experience at working towards more than one refraining-based self-discipline goal and you have had some success in this area;
   (c) your confidence level at working towards self-discipline across the board is quite high;
   (d) you can apply general concepts to specific situations and enjoy doing so;

(e)   you prefer the idea of striving towards refraining-based self-discipline across the board to working on one or more than one (but not all) refraining-based self-discipline goals at a time.

Once you have decided on a particular approach to addressing two or more refraining-based self-discipline goals, you can always change tack later. For example, if you have decided to approach your problems one at a time and you have been successful with this approach, then you might try to tackle two further problems at once, for example, if what you have learned from achieving your first goal is applicable to these other problems. If changing tack does not work, you can always revert to the strategy that has brought you success.

An example of striving for self-discipline across the board

You may be wondering what is involved in addressing all your refraining-based self-discipline goals at once and striving for self-discipline across the board. To illustrate this let me discuss the case of Terence. When he came to see me, Terence had just had a thorough physical examination and had been told by his physician that he had to make several drastic changes to his lifestyle if he was to avoid developing serious medical problems. This proved to be a wake-up call for Terence, who up to that point had enjoyed an epicurean life-style based on the well-known principle: 'Eat, drink and be merry, for tomorrow you might die.' Well, the latter part of this aphorism was proving a real possibility and this prompted Terence to seek my help in making immediate and drastic changes to the way he approached life.

Terence wanted to achieve the following refraining-based self-discipline goals:

- Stop smoking.
- Abstain from alcohol.
- Cut out high carbohydrate and high fat foods.
- Stop taking drugs.
- Stop gambling.
- Go to bed at 10.30 p.m. instead of staying up until 4.00 a.m. playing computer games.

I also helped Terence set goals based on initiating self-disciplined behaviour, but I will focus here on what he did to refrain from engaging in self-undisciplined behaviour across the board.

Terence met most of the criteria that I outlined above, indicating why an across-the-board approach to refraining-based self-discipline should be considered.

- Terence decided to adopt this approach because he was told that he had to make drastic and immediate changes to his lifestyle, a lifestyle that was endangering his life. He therefore had a very good reason to adopt this approach.
- He had some successful experience in the past at giving up smoking and abstaining from alcohol, but did not maintain it because, in his words, 'I thought I could smoke and drink and get away with it.'
- His confidence level concerning being successful at implementing an across-the-board approach to self-discipline was high since, again in his words, 'When I put my mind to something, I am generally successful at it and the fact that I may well die if I don't change my ways concentrates the mind wonderfully!'
- Finally, Terence was adept at applying general concepts to specific self-discipline threatening situations. He was a high-flying management consultant well used to utilizing general principles in specific management situations.

Having decided to abstain from smoking, drinking, eating unhealthy foods, drug-taking, gambling and playing computer games late at night, Terence carried out a self-monitoring exercise on his urges to engage in these activities. He discovered that his urges to engage in these activities occurred (1) when he was bored, (2) when he failed to have his desires met in other areas of his life and (3) when he was with friends who encouraged him to join them in drinking, smoking and taking drugs. Terence saw clearly that he was engaging in pleasurable but ultimately life-threatening activities as a way of not experiencing the disturbed feelings he would have felt if he was bored, did not get what he wanted, said 'no' to his friends and abstained from engaging in these activities.

Here I will concentrate on how I helped Terence deal with boredom, desire deprivation and the urges themselves.

Terence dealt with his boredom tolerance in two ways. First, every time he experienced boredom he challenged his demand that he had to get rid of boredom quickly, and second, to that end he practised staying with feeling bored while showing himself that he could stand feeling this way although he would never like it. Only when he raised his tolerance for feeling bored would he engage in non-harmful activities that were interesting and involving for him. It is important to note that if Terence immediately engaged in such involving activities as soon as he became bored, he would neither gain the experience of raising his tolerance for boredom nor have the opportunity to develop his non-dogmatic preference concerning boredom (i.e. 'I would like to get rid of boredom straight away, but I don't have to do so').

Terence practised his healthy beliefs concerning boredom in areas where he would previously have engaged in the very behaviours that were now posing a real threat to his life. As he said to me once: 'Experiencing boredom won't kill me, but engaging in the behaviour I developed so that I wouldn't feel bored very well might!'

Terence dealt with the issue of desire deprivation in a similar way. First, he showed himself that while it is nice to have his desires met immediately (e.g. winning a contract at work, a girl accepting his offer of a date), it is not necessary for him to get what he wants. He also showed himself that while being deprived of what he wants immediately is difficult to tolerate, it is tolerable and it is definitely worth it for him to tolerate because doing so means that he is less likely to engage in activities that threaten his well-being. Having consolidated this rational belief about being deprived of his immediate desire, instead of engaging in pleasurable but self-undisciplined activities Terence pursued alternative desires that were more within his control, such as writing poetry and keeping a diary for his young nephews recording his experiences developing greater self-discipline and exercise.

Terence dealt with his urges to engage in self-undisciplined behaviour by showing himself that just because he experiences an urge to engage in self-undisciplined behaviour, he doesn't have to act on this urge, and if he carries on with his everyday activities while experiencing such urges they will diminish in intensity over time after immediately and briefly increasing in intensity once he does not satisfy them.

Notice from the above that Terence did the following:

- He challenged his irrational beliefs about boredom and practised his alternative, developing rational beliefs while feeling bored.
- He challenged his irrational beliefs about not having his desires met and practised new rational beliefs while experiencing this deprivation.
- He challenged irrational beliefs about his urges to act in self-undisciplined ways and practised thinking rationally while letting himself experience these urges without acting on them.

In all these three areas, Terence referred to his more conceptual, general irrational beliefs and used these to identify and challenge specific versions of these beliefs in relevant specific situations. Additionally, he referred to his general rational beliefs to formulate specific versions of these beliefs in the same situations, which he then practised while acting in ways that would help to strengthen them and while refraining from engaging in the self-undisciplined behaviour from which he wanted to abstain.

I also mentioned that Terence came under pressure to engage in self-undisciplined activities from some of his friends. In the following chapter, I will discuss how to deal with such pressures, as well as how you can elicit support and encouragement from others as you pursue your self-discipline goals.

Part 5
Keep going

Once you have achieved your self-discipline goals, is that the end of the story? Far from it! Although it is hard to address your self-discipline problems and work towards your goals, it is perhaps harder to maintain the gains that you have made. In the final part of this book, I will first discuss the role that other people play in helping you to maintain your gains or in wittingly or unwittingly attempting to sabotage your efforts, and what you can do to encourage them in the former and discourage them in the latter. Then, I will consider how to identify and deal productively with the most common obstacles to keeping going along the path to continuing self-discipline.

11

The role of other people in developing and maintaining self-discipline

Although developing and maintaining self-discipline is ultimately a matter for you alone as an individual, other people in your life can make a great deal of difference in helping you to reach and maintain your self-discipline goals or hindering you in this process. I will begin this chapter by discussing how other people can help you to develop and maintain self-discipline and how you can encourage them in this regard. Then, I will discuss how people unwittingly or wittingly try to sabotage you in your efforts to develop and maintain self-discipline and how to deal with this if and when it occurs. Please note that, in my discussion, I will not discuss the role of formal therapists in helping or hindering you as you negotiate your way through the difficulties, since this falls outside my remit in writing a book for you to use on your own.

Other people as a helpful resource

As I have said, ultimately you are responsible for developing and maintaining self-discipline, but almost always other people are involved, for better or worse, in this process. In this part of the chapter, I will discuss the things that people do that are generally helpful to you as you strive to acquire and maintain self-discipline, and then I will show you what you can do to elicit their help.

How others can help you in the process of developing and maintaining self-discipline

There are basically four ways in which other people can be helpful to you as you strive to develop and maintain self-discipline.

People can offer support and encouragement

As I have stressed several times in this book, pursuing self-discipline goals is a difficult process, and maintaining self-discipline is perhaps even harder. Given this, you can do with all the help you can get from other people. Having people in your life who will support and encourage you during this process, and particularly when the going gets tough, can be especially helpful. Such support and encouragement can take many forms. Here are a number of examples. Remember one thing, though, as you read this list. People vary enormously in what they find supportive and encouraging. Your job is to discover what you personally find supportive and encouraging, and to seek out people in your life who will provide you with these ingredients. These may be significant people in your life or people who are going through the same process of dealing with self-discipline problems as you (as in Alcoholics Anonymous).

Support and encouragement may come from

- being told that your progress matters to the person;
- being told that you can do it;
- being encouraged to stay with your goals when the going gets tough;
- having someone to talk to for support when the going gets tough, either in person, by phone or live over the internet (as I mentioned earlier in this book, this is a major reason why Alcoholics Anonymous works for a lot of people);
- having someone to discuss your problems with (these can be problems related or unrelated to the area of self-discipline);
- having someone to turn to when you need company;
- having someone empathize with you as you pursue your goals, and particularly showing you that he or she understands how hard it is and how lapsing occasionally is to be expected.

As I have already discussed, in Alcoholics Anonymous each person has a sponsor. This person is someone who is further along the road in pursuing the 12 steps of the AA programme than the person being sponsored, and has the experience of the struggles people experience in achieving and maintaining sobriety. This means that if you are in the AA fellowship, the support and encouragement that you receive from your sponsor is underpinned by real experience of what you are going through. While some people value support and encouragement from wherever it comes, others only value and are helped by these ingredients when they are offered by those who have been through what they are going through.

It is helpful to build up a support network of people who can encourage you through the process of acquiring and maintaining self-discipline. As you develop your support network, ask yourself whether or not it matters to you if the people offering you support and encouragement have already been through a similar process, and choose accordingly.

People can serve as your therapeutic aide

A second way that a person can help you is as a therapeutic aide. This is perhaps a more formal role than the one that I have just discussed, but not as formal as the role of therapist, which, as I said at the beginning of this chapter, falls outside the scope of this book. The job of a therapeutic aide is to help you apply the principles of any self-help programme that you are following. To do this the person needs to learn about the skills that you will be learning and how they can be applied to the acquisition and maintenance of self-discipline. The person may or may not have used these skills in his or her own life, but this is not the crucial issue. What is central is that the person knows how they should be used and can help you to use them in your own life.

Jeremy's example

Jeremy asked one of his friends, Ken, to serve as his therapeutic aide. He chose Ken because Ken was interested in psychology and had served as a volunteer counsellor at the Nightline telephone counselling service when they were both at university. Jeremy was given six sessions with a CBT therapist at his local GP practice who was using a similar approach to self-discipline to the one outlined in this book. During his brief therapy, Jeremy was asked by his counsellor to carry out a variety of tasks, including completing forms focused on:

- self-monitoring;
- identifying the self-defeating thoughts and beliefs that preceded instances of self-indiscipline;
- challenging these self-defeating thoughts and beliefs;
- dealing with urges.

Each form had precise instructions, and Ken used these to check Jeremy's homework before his next therapy session. So successful was Ken in his role as therapy aide that Jeremy was able to space out his six sessions over six months while he consolidated the skills and the gains that he made with Ken's help. Ken was careful to hand the reins over to Jeremy as the latter became more adept at his CBT skills, and this is a core talent of an effective therapy aide: to help a person like Jeremy become his own therapist rather than serving as therapist for him.

You can develop self-discipline with like-minded people

One of the advantages of group therapy over individual therapy is that it provides a context for people to gain a sense of 'being in the same boat', as it were, in the journey towards psychological growth, rather than sailing in the boat alone. This is another reason why helping communities focused on self-discipline, like Alcoholics Anonymous and WeightWatchers, are helpful to people. Both of these organizations, and others that have been developed in their image, offer a helping context where everybody is working towards common goals.

This sense of community can be tremendously helpful to some people and irrelevant to others. If you think that you will be aided in the development and maintenance of self-discipline by working towards such goals alongside others who are also working towards similar goals, then either join an existing community or set up your own self-help group. Michael, a university student, tried working on his own and with an individual counsellor to overcome his chronic procrastination, both to no avail. Then, realizing that he might find it helpful to work with other like-minded people to become more self-disciplined, he set up a small self-help group designed to help people address their problems with procrastination. He called the group SWOOSH after the Nike logo, which was associated at that time with the phrase: 'Just do it.' While a number of people joined the group and quickly left (remember that such self-helping communities are not for everyone), a small caucus of people remained with the group over the course of their university career and attributed their success at university in no small part to the self-help group established by Michael. Michael himself benefited from the group and said later that he felt a sense of obligation to be a role model for the group (see below), saying: 'If the founder of the group kept procrastinating, what message would that convey to others, both existing members and those thinking of joining?'

While existing self-help communities like Alcoholics Anonymous, WeightWatchers and SMART Recovery (an organization designed to help people address their problems with alcohol, based on similar principles to those outlined in this book) have their own methodologies, if you are thinking about establishing a self-help community you can either use a book such as this one as a guiding framework or you can develop your own materials based on what group members find helpful. Remember, though, that for those who find such communities helpful the sense of 'being in the same boat' is more important than the methodology used by the communities.

People can serve as role models for you

Another way in which people can help you in the self-discipline process is to inspire you with their own example. If you are inspired by how others have overcome their self-discipline problems and maintained self-discipline over time, then by all means use their example to help you along your own path to self-discipline.

There are plenty of examples in the newspapers and magazines of how people have made great strides in developing self-discipline. These examples are usually of refraining-based self-discipline, where the stories recounted are of how people have lost a great deal of weight, become sober after years of alcohol abuse and foresworn drug-taking and gambling after losing everything they had, including their families. Often the stories that make the press are either of celebrities or of ordinary people who have achieved considerable self-discipline goals (e.g. losing an enormous amount of weight). These stories follow a similar pattern. First, they give a potted history of the person concerned, often focusing on adversities he or she suffered growing up, such as abuse, bullying at school or falling in with the wrong crowd. Second, they explain how the person turned to a life of self-indiscipline to cope with these problems or as a way of keeping in with the crowd. Third, they outline, often in graphic detail, the negative effects of self-indiscipline on the life of the person. Finally, they show how the person – often only after reaching rock bottom – turned to some organization or treatment community and achieved stunning results, turning his or her life around. There are almost always 'before' and 'after' pictures which show the difference between the person before self-discipline and after self-discipline. Particularly common are pictures of the person grossly overweight and now super-slim, since these images show, in dramatic form, what can be achieved.

The advantage of these stories, in my view, is to show that human beings are capable of overcoming adversity and performing great feats of self-discipline, and as such they may inspire you along the lines of 'If they can do it, so can I.' However, since such stories are dramatic they do not, in general, show that it is often more difficult maintaining one's self-discipline goals over time than it is to achieve them in the first place. Stories of how people, particularly ordinary people, have maintained self-discipline years after reaching their self-discipline goals are not common in the press, because they lack the drama of the stories recounting how people have achieved great goals of self-discipline in the first place. One exception to this, particularly when the subject is a celebrity, is when the person has achieved self-discipline, has maintained it for a while, and has then fallen off the wagon before climbing back on again.

For those of you who are inspired by these stories and find some of their subjects good role models, you can learn from their example and particularly from their mistakes. However, if you prefer to know your role models personally, then look for people who have experienced similar problems and have maintained self-discipline over time. It is perhaps better if your role model has experienced some lapses in the maintenance phase since, as I will discuss in the final chapter, lapses in the maintenance phase of self-discipline are quite common. As such, you may be able to learn from their experiences and avoid making the same mistakes as they did, although in all probability you will make some of your own. The important point here, as I will discuss in Chapter 12, is that lapses can be learned from and do not have to lead to relapse.

Finally, if your role model is prepared to mentor you in your quest to achieve and maintain your self-discipline goals, then you will have the benefit of his or her experience and ongoing advice when you need it. Good sponsors in AA serve this dual function. However, it is important that you don't become dependent on your mentor but use his or her experiences and advice to become your own self-discipline counsellor.

What you can do to elicit help from others

So far in this chapter, I have argued that people can be helpful to you in the field of self-discipline by offering you support and encouragement, by serving as a kind of therapeutic aide, by working with you as you both strive towards self-discipline and by serving as a role model and advice-giver. But what do you need to do to elicit help from people? Here is what I suggest.

- Work out for yourself the type of help you need from other people.
- Target the person or people that you think can be helpful to you.
- Admit to them that you have problems with self-discipline and what your goals are.
- Tell them what help you want from them and ask them if they are able and willing to provide such help.
- If they agree, work out the practicalities of such help, in particular how best to contact them for help and when to do so.

When other people are unhelpful

However, not all people will be helpful to you as you work towards your self-discipline goals. In this part of the chapter, I will outline the ways in which people may be unhelpful to you and what you can do when you encounter such people.

Witting vs. unwitting sabotage

When other people are unhelpful to you, it may be that they are serving to sabotage your efforts unwittingly or wittingly. I will begin by discussing how to respond when people are unwittingly being unhelpful to you. However, I first want to make an important point about language. You will note throughout what follows that I talk about others unwittingly or wittingly *attempting* to sabotage you rather than them sabotaging you. This is very deliberate. I firmly hold that other people do not sabotage you. If, as a result of their unhelpful behaviour, you act in a self-undisciplined manner, then you are responsible for that behaviour; they are not. They are responsible for their own behaviour. Remember this and you will refrain from blaming others for your own behaviour, a practice which, if engaged in, will decidedly interfere with you learning from incidents of your self-undisciplined behaviour in the face of sabotage attempts from others.

When people attempt to sabotage you unwittingly

Unwitting attempts at sabotage occur when people act in ways that make it more difficult for you to act in self-disciplined ways because they do not know that you are working towards self-discipline goals. A typical example occurs when you are on a low calorie diet and you visit someone who has made a high calorie meal, not knowing that by doing so he or she is making it harder for you to remain with your diet (harder, you will note – not impossible!).

The obvious thing to do here is to tell people in advance that you are addressing your self-discipline problems and to ask them to help you achieve and maintain your goals. In the above example, this would mean that, on receiving the invitation, you tell the person that you are on a low calorie diet and ask if he or she will help you by preparing for you a low calorie meal, perhaps even being specific about what you can eat, since people's ideas about what constitutes a low calorie meal often do not accord with reality. In order to do this, you will have to challenge any irrational beliefs that impede such self-interest. Here are a few examples of such self-impeding thoughts, the irrational beliefs that underpin them and how they impact on behaviour, rational alternatives to these beliefs and how these lead to different behaviours.

Thought	'I don't want to be a nuisance'
Irrational belief	'I must not put them to any trouble'
Action based on irrational belief	Don't tell them about food preferences
Rational belief	'I don't want to put them to any trouble, but in life there is no reason why this must not happen from time to time. Since I want to achieve my goals, I will do so on this occasion.'
Action based on rational belief	Tell them about my food preferences
Thought	'Asking for what I want may appear selfish'
Irrational belief	'I must not appear selfish'
Action based on irrational belief	Don't tell them about food preferences

| *Rational belief* | 'I don't want to appear selfish, but I am not immune from being seen in this way. If I am seen in this way by asking for certain foods, that doesn't make me selfish, and if I don't look after myself, nobody will' |
| *Action based on rational belief* | Tell them about my food preferences |

When people wittingly attempt to sabotage you

When you tell other people that you are working towards self-discipline goals and ask them to help you, but they act in ways that again make it more difficult for you to act in a self-disciplined manner, then they are wittingly attempting to sabotage your efforts. Such witting attempts may occur for different reasons (e.g. people may not take your self-disciplined efforts seriously or they may envy you your success). The main point is not why they try to sabotage you, but how you can best respond to these sabotage attempts. I will now outline some useful responses to such sabotage attempts.

Use their sabotage efforts as a way of strengthening your self-discipline muscles   When people wittingly try to sabotage your attempts to engage in self-disciplined behaviour, you can view it as an opportunity to strengthen your self-discipline muscles in the face of adversity. The most frequent way that people attempt to sabotage you is to tempt you to engage in self-undisciplined behaviour and encourage you to feel bad if you don't engage in it. For example, Colin, who we met earlier in the book, wanted to address his procrastination and made progress in doing so using the cognitive–behavioural methods outlined in this book. However, two of his friends, Andy and Mike, frequently knocked on his study door inviting him to join them down the pub for drinks, and when he said 'no' told him he was turning into a nerd for studying rather than partying. Colin decided to use these attempts at sabotaging him as an opportunity to practise rational thinking and constructive action in the face of such temptation, for he admitted to himself that he enjoyed his friends' company and regarded an evening spent with them as vastly more enjoyable than studying. Despite this, Colin rehearsed the following beliefs:

- 'It would be fun going out tonight, but I don't need to have fun right now. I can tolerate the deprivation.'
- 'I am not a nerd even if Andy and Mike think I am. I am an ordinary human being and I recognize that to get my degree I need to put work before play.'

- 'I don't need Andy and Mike's approval even though I value it.'

Having rehearsed these beliefs, Colin said 'no' and kept saying 'no' until he was ready to go out, which was after he had achieved a set amount of work.

You can follow Colin's example and use the witting attempts of others to sabotage your self-disciplined efforts by staying on course behaviourally, while challenging the irrational beliefs that would otherwise lead you to give in to the sabotage and practising your developing rational beliefs instead.

Assert yourself When people wittingly try to sabotage you when you are attempting to act in a self-disciplined manner, then a powerful way of responding is by asserting yourself. Assertion, in this context, can involve a number of components, such as the following:

- Say 'no' to offers from others to engage in self-undisciplined behaviour.
- Do not agree with any pejorative remarks made by others when you say 'no', but do not try to dissuade them.
- Ask others to agree to refrain from inviting you to engage in self-undisciplined behaviour.

Here is how Colin used these steps when Andy and Mike attempted once again to sabotage his studying.

Andy: Hey, Colin, we're going out for a beer. Do you fancy coming along? (1)

Colin: No, mate, I've got work to do. (2)

Mike: Come on, mate, you can do the work later. Don't be a teacher's pet. (3)

Colin: I am not a teacher's pet. (4)

Andy: No, Mike, Colin's more like a boring nerd. Man, you used to be such fun. (5)

Colin: I am still fun, but fun now comes after work. Can we agree that you will respect my decision to study before partying? (6)

Andy: We will talk about that when you come to your senses. Mike, let's leave Mr Swot with his books. (7)

In this example you will see that Colin uses the components of assertion as follows.

- He says 'no' to Mike's offer to engage in self-undisciplined behaviour (response 2).
- He actively disagrees with both Mike's and Andy's pejorative remarks, but does not try to dissuade them (responses 4 and 6).

- He asks Andy and Mike to agree to refrain from inviting him out when he is working (response 6).

Notice that Colin's attempt to elicit agreement from Andy and Mike that they will not sabotage him in future is not successful. This is an important point. The purpose of assertion in this context is not to persuade others to desist from sabotage, although if they agree to do so and follow through on this that is a bonus. The purpose of assertion is to make your position clear and to continue to act in a self-disciplined way whether or not others continue to attempt to sabotage you. If you want to learn more about assertion, you might find it helpful to consult a book that I wrote with my colleague, Daniel Constantinou, entitled *Assertiveness: Step by Step* (Sheldon Press, 2004).

Confront your saboteurs   Another way to deal with people who attempt to sabotage you wittingly is to confront them about it. Confrontation seeks to bring to the other's attention that you know that he (in this case) is trying to sabotage you and that you want to know why he is doing it as well as seeking to persuade him to stop.

Confrontation can be a powerful but high-risk strategy, in that it brings things to a head. It may lead the person to stop sabotaging you, but it may result in people increasing their sabotage attempts or even ending their relationship with you, something that you may not want to happen. It is for this reason that I recommend that you use this approach after you have asserted yourself and it has failed to stop others' sabotage attempts.

Here is how Colin eventually confronted Andy and Mike when they continued their sabotage attempts after Colin asserted himself and requested them to stop.

Mike: Hey, Colin, coming out to the pub with us?

Colin: No, mate, I have some studying to do.

Andy: Oh come on, Colin, that's the same thing you said yesterday. There's a great band playing tonight. They are right up your street.

Colin: No thanks. Maybe I'll join you after I have finished this essay.

Mike: OK, Mr Swot, maybe later.

Colin: You know, you guys, this is bugging me. I told you that I'm going to put studying before partying and asked you to respect that, but you don't. Why are you trying to sabotage me?

Andy: What do you mean, sabotage you?

Colin: Real friends respect what their friends want to do, even if they don't like it. I am asking you both to respect my wishes. Please do that.

Mike: OK, Mr Swot ... we get the message. We won't bother you again. Right, Andy?

Andy: Right. Ciao, Colin.

In Colin's case, confrontation brought things to a head but resulted in Andy and Mike saying that they would leave him alone, which they did for a while before making it up with Colin later and respecting his wishes. Please note, however, that confrontation may lead to the permanent dissolution of relationships.

Offer to help them with their self-discipline problems   It is quite likely, when other people attempt to sabotage your self-discipline efforts, that they have problems with self-discipline themselves. It may sound strange, but one way of responding to the sabotage efforts of such people is to offer to help them to address their self-discipline problems. If by chance they agree to your offer, then you have disarmed the 'enemy', as it were, and have recruited them to 'your side'. Indeed, if they agree to your offer then they may join a helping community such as the ones I discussed in the first part of this chapter.

If Colin had attempted this strategy, this is how he might have done so:

Mike: Hey, Colin, coming out to the pub with us?

Colin: No, mate, I have some studying to do.

Andy: Oh come on, Colin, that's the same thing you said yesterday. There's a great band playing tonight. They are right up your street.

Colin: Hey, you two, have you lost interest in getting a degree?

Mike: No, why?

Colin: Because you are acting like that.

Andy: No, we'll be all right. It's party today, study tomorrow.

Colin: Well, that's a high-risk strategy, in my view. Why not join me in my study first, party later strategy. We can still have a real good time. We can all work together on this, get our degrees and still have a great time. What do you say?

The important thing to remember here is that Colin can continue to pursue his self-discipline goals whether or not Andy and Mike accept his offer of help. And the same point applies to you. By all means offer to help your saboteurs. But keep focused on your self-discipline goals whether or not they accept your offer.

Develop relationships with people who are self-disciplined

If your saboteurs continue their attempts at sabotage despite your various attempts to dissuade them, then avoid them if you can and ignore them if you can't. In the latter case, keep focused on your self-discipline goals in the face of their ongoing attempts at sabotage. Try not to engage them in further attempts at dissuasion since these are unlikely to work. Instead, develop relationships with people who are self-disciplined. If you do this you will be around people who share your values and will encourage you in your own self-disciplined efforts, or who at least are not likely to discourage you from acting in a self-undisciplined manner.

There is one exception to this last point. Some people who are successful in their own self-disciplined efforts will try, in subtle ways, to encourage you to fail in yours. They need you to fail so that they can feel superior to you or so that they can help you. Whatever the motivation, if you encounter such sabotage among people who are self-disciplined then you can use one or more of the strategies that I discussed above.

Once you have achieved your self-discipline goals with or without the help of others, then you still have to work to maintain your self-disciplined behaviour, and it is to this subject that I turn in the following and final chapter of this book.

12

Maintain self-discipline

Many people who have succeeded in reaching their self-discipline goals have attested to the fact that it is even harder to maintain self-discipline, hence the Mark Twain quote: 'Giving up smoking is easy, I've done it hundreds of times.' So, to a large extent, giving up smoking, for example, is just a first step – an important step to be sure – but a first step nevertheless. The question becomes how to stay stopped.

In this chapter, then, I will discuss how you might develop self-discipline as a way of life in those areas of your life where you have decided to be self-disciplined.

Continue practising good habits of thinking and behaving

Ross Perot, who twice stood as a candidate for the US presidency, made a telling point about the difficulty of self-discipline maintenance. He said: 'Something in human nature causes us to start slacking off at our moment of greatest accomplishment. As you become successful, you will need a great deal of self-discipline not to lose your sense of balance, humility and commitment.'

Let's suppose that through hard work and self-discipline you have reached your target weight. According to Perot you may well experience a tendency to slacken off in terms of effort, a sense of feeling pleased with yourself and a diminution of your commitment to maintain your weight. You may also think that you have earned the right to go off the rails a little. If you do experience these things – which may be a natural response to achieving goals that you have worked hard to achieve – it does not follow that you have to act on them. Thus, you can still keep acting in a self-disciplined manner (with modifications in the weight control area so that you maintain your weight rather than continue to lose it) even though you may experience the urge to slacken off.

You may plan to make certain changes to your self-discipline regime once you have achieved your goals (as I discuss later in this chapter) but, by and large, the main thing you need to do once you have achieved your goals is to continue the rational thinking and constructive behaviour that you employed to achieve your goals in the first place.

Apart from the natural tendency to slacken off once you have initially achieved your goals, there are other reasons why you might not continue to think rationally and act constructively in the same manner in the maintenance phase as you did in the goal achievement phase. Let me list two main reasons and how to deal with them.

The demand that maintaining self-discipline should be easier than its development and its associated LFT belief

Having achieved your self-discipline goals through hard work, you may think that maintaining self-discipline must be easier than achieving it in the first place. Dogmatically believing that it must be easier to maintain self-discipline than it was to achieve it means that when you discover that it is not easier – that indeed it is as difficult or in some ways even more difficult – you quickly get discouraged, because you think that you cannot bear to make an ongoing commitment to act in a disciplined manner when it is not easier and because you see a life full of effort and discipline, with no joy. In short, your dogmatic demand and associated low frustration tolerance (LFT) belief about the ease or otherwise of continued self-discipline leads you to a biased view of the future, with no room for joy.

In order to get things into perspective, you need to challenge and change your dogmatic demand and LFT belief, as detailed above, and replace it and act on a flexible and non-extreme alternative. In doing this you need to show yourself the following:

- that if maintaining self-discipline is as difficult or even more difficult than achieving self-discipline goals in the first place, then that is reality and it does not have to be any different even if it is undesirable;
- that just because you want maintenance of self-discipline to be easier than its acquisition, this does not mean that you have to get what you want;
- that it may be a struggle to put up with ongoing effort and difficulty as you strive to maintain your self-discipline, but it is tolerable and it is definitely worth it to you to tolerate it. If in doubt, review your self-discipline goals and the values that underpinned them that you identified when you decided to address your problems of self-indiscipline (see Chapter 3).

When you think rationally about the ongoing difficulty of maintaining self-discipline, then you will see that you can integrate putting up with this difficulty into your everyday life and see that doing so does not preclude you from having fun. I hope you can see then that developing a flexible, non-extreme attitude about the difficulty of maintaining self-discipline is far more likely to encourage you to maintain it than your dogmatic extreme attitude towards such difficulty.

Overconfidence

As the quote from Ross Perot shows, when you achieve your self-discipline goals you tend to lose your humility. One of the ways in which this becomes evident is in an overconfident attitude about maintaining your gains. When you are overconfident, you make one or both of two errors:

- You underestimate the difficulties that you will encounter as you work to maintain your self-discipline, having initially achieved your goals.
- You overestimate how easy you will find it to deal with the difficulties that you do encounter.

In either case, your overconfidence tends to lead you to slacken off, with the results that you will increase the chances that you will experience numerous lapses and will ultimately relapse. So what can you do to deal with overconfidence? I recommend the following:

- Acknowledge that you are experiencing overconfidence rather than confidence about the task of maintaining self-discipline. If you were confident you would have faith in your ability to handle the difficulties to be faced in the maintenance phase, but you would not overestimate that ability, nor would you underestimate those difficulties to be faced. Overconfidence involves overestimating one's ability and/or underestimating the difficulties.
- Recognize that you have done well to achieve your self-discipline goals and acknowledge that the ability on which your achievements were based will serve you well as you strive to maintain your self-discipline. However, it does not follow that you will find dealing with maintaining self-discipline easier than it is.
- Resolve to use the same level of commitment to maintain your self-discipline goals as you did when you were striving to achieve them, and resolve to use increased commitment at times when the going gets tougher than expected in the maintenance phase.

Develop a non-perfectionistic attitude about maintaining your gains

It is important that you understand that the process of change is rarely smooth and that you will frequently take two steps forward and one step back, or even one step forward and two steps back! This is true even when you have initially achieved your self-discipline goals. When these setbacks are small and when they occur in the context of your general progress, they are best described as lapses. However, when you experience a significant setback this is perhaps better described as a relapse. I will deal with relapse and relapse prevention presently.

Having a perfectionistic attitude towards progress in the maintenance phase of self-discipline means that you believe that you must not lapse, and if you do it's terrible and you might as well give up if you cannot sustain self-discipline perfectly. It is important that you dispute this pernicious idea, as it will quickly lead you back to a self-undisciplined lifestyle. The idea is:

- unrealistic (if such a natural law existed that you must not lapse, you wouldn't be able to lapse since the law would prevent you. A moment's thought belies the realism of this idea: as a human it is always possible for you to lapse as you are fallible, which means prone to error);
- illogical (it does not logically follow that because you would rather not lapse, therefore you must not);
- dysfunctional (as I have already shown you, as long as you believe that you must not lapse and you do so, then you are far more likely to give up continuing to be self-disciplined than if you hold a flexible belief about lapsing).

Such a flexible belief takes the following form: 'I would prefer not to lapse, but I am not immune from doing so. If I do lapse, it's unfortunate, but not terrible.' This non-perfectionistic attitude is:

- realistic (it is both true that you would prefer not to lapse and also true that you are not immune from doing so);
- logical (the idea that you are not immune from lapsing follows logically from the idea that you would prefer not to lapse);
- functional (it leads to good results in that you won't give up at the first sign of a lapse).

Put this non-perfectionistic attitude about maintaining your gains into practice as much as you can and it will help you to learn from lapsing and to maintain self-discipline.

Deal with lapses

It is important that you accept your lapsing as normal – as something that happens to almost all people who have achieved their self-discipline goals – so you can see it as part of your human fallibility. Challenge the idea that while others can lapse, you must not do so. Acknowledge that even *you* are not immune from occasionally backsliding. In this way, you will feel disappointed but not ashamed when you act in a self-undisciplined manner. Not feeling ashamed about your lapse, you will be open to seeking help from others rather than dealing with the lapses on your own.

When you lapse, look at your self-undisciplined behaviour as bad and unfortunate, rather than terrible, and accept yourself for engaging in this behaviour. Rate your lapsing as bad, not yourself, and then look at the lapse and the factors that occasioned it so that you can learn from this and similar experiences. In this respect you can use the ABC framework that I outlined earlier to understand the lapse, challenge the irrational beliefs that underpinned the lapse and rehearse the alternative rational beliefs.

Lightly or 'intellectually' rehearsing your new rational beliefs won't help very much or convince you for very long. Rather, rehearse them in a strong and vigorous manner and do so many times. Thus, you can powerfully go over such rational beliefs as: 'I do not need what I want!' and 'I can tolerate not acting on my urge, no matter how strong it is!' until you are really convinced of them and, in common parlance, really feel them in your gut.

Practise relapse prevention

'Relapse prevention' is a term which originated in work with the addictions, to highlight the fact that relapse often occurs and that a concerted effort to help yourself prevent relapse is frequently necessary. A major part of relapse prevention involves you becoming aware of a variety of vulnerability factors. Vulnerability factors are factors which can occur in your external or internal world and render you vulnerable to acting in a self-undisciplined manner.

Let's take dealing with alcohol problems as an example. External vulnerability factors include the sight and smell of alcohol, other people drinking and TV adverts for drink, while internal vulnerability factors include the following:

- styles of thinking (e.g. thinking of all the positive aspects of drinking alcohol);
- behaviour patterns (deliberately walking past pubs and bars when you are not ready to do so);
- emotional responses (positive feelings associated with drink and negative feelings which in the past you have extinguished through alcohol);
- urges to drink.

All of these serve as invitations for you to drink.

In relapse prevention, you take each problem on your problem list and identify the set of internal and external circumstances in which you might experience a relapse. Be as specific as you can be when you identify relapse-triggering events and the irrational beliefs you hold about such events. In particular, identify any vulnerable feelings which may discourage you from using the techniques you have learned in this book.

Then, imagine that you are experiencing such a vulnerable feeling or entering into a situation in which you may be vulnerable to relapse, and use your rational thinking skills to prevent the situation leading to relapse. You might do this by using imagery techniques or self-help forms. After you have successfully coped with your vulnerability factors in imagination, you can then seek them out in reality so that you can gain experience of using your developing rational thinking skills in real-life situations.

Ways of approaching your vulnerability factors

As you seek out the vulnerability factors to gain the experience of dealing with them productively, you can do so in one of three ways:

1 *Fully and quickly*: this approach has the potential of bringing about the most change in the quickest possible time, but you may well find this 'full-on' approach to confronting your vulnerability factors overwhelming.
2 *Slowly and gradually*: with this approach you minimize discomfort as you approach your vulnerability factors, but there is little challenge involved. In adopting this approach you may also unwittingly reinforce your LFT beliefs about discomfort.
3 *Challenging, but not overwhelming*: here, you approach your vulnerability factors in a way that is challenging for you, but not overwhelming to you. This is the approach that is most likely to be effective for you and is the one that I recommend most of my clients use in dealing with their vulnerability factors in the maintenance phase of self-discipline.

Accepting yourself for your failures will help you learn from these failures

It is particularly important for you to accept yourself if you fail to use your rational thinking skills in real-life vulnerable situations and experience a relapse. Doing so will help you to get back on the self-discipline track. When you think rationally about relapse you can more easily learn from the experience than when you think irrationally about it. Thinking rationally in this area will enable you to see that every setback is a useful learning experience if you can remain sufficiently open-minded rather than self-depreciating about these setbacks.

Deal with your fear of relapse

Some people fear relapse and think that even a slight act of self-indiscipline means relapse. The roots of such a fear are founded on a dogmatic attitude towards self-control (as discussed in Chapter 6). Thus, if you believe that you have to be in control of your behaviour at all times and you begin to act in a self-undisciplined manner, you will get anxious and think that this small instance of self-indiscipline will inevitably end in a complete self-indiscipline relapse. In some people, this fear means that they avoid doing anything or going anywhere where they might engage in the smallest act of self-indiscipline. In other people, when they engage in a small act of self-indiscipline they think that they have 'blown it' and that since relapse is inevitable they might as well get it over with.

The way to deal with the fear of relapse is twofold:

1 Change your dogmatic attitude towards any lapse in self-discipline.
2 Take the horror out of relapse.

I will show you how to do this by referring to the case of Miriam, who feared relapse with her diet. Miriam had done very well and had lost two stone on a low calorie diet which she was advised to follow by her GP for health reasons. She was very rigorous in following guidelines similar to those outlined in this book and achieved her weight goals without any lapses. It was when she had to modify her diet to maintain her weight that her fear emerged. When Miriam modified her diet, on the first day of doing so she ate too much and, instead of treating this as a lapse to learn from, she panicked and went back to her previous weight-losing diet. Her doctor referred her to me for counselling since she had lost too much but was fearful of returning to the weight-maintenance diet.

Change your dogmatic attitude towards any lapse in self-discipline

I helped Miriam identify the dogmatic attitude that underpinned her fear. It was: 'I must not eat more than I am allowed and it will be terrible if I do.' Then I helped her develop a flexible alternative to this belief, namely: 'I would prefer not to eat more than I am allowed, but that doesn't mean that I must not do it. If I eat more, that would be unfortunate but not terrible.' I helped Miriam see that her dogmatic belief and the awfulizing belief that stemmed from it are false, illogical and dysfunctional, and that her non-dogmatic preference and the anti-awfulizing belief that stemmed from it are true, logical and functional.

Importantly, I helped Miriam to see that when she held her irrational belief about experiencing a lapse in self-discipline, then she would overestimate how much self-control she would lose. By contrast, if she held a rational belief about experiencing a lapse, then she would keep the extent of the lapse in perspective.

In order to internalize her rational belief, I encouraged her to practise it while deliberately eating more than she planned on a number of occasions and while visiting places which she had previously avoided because she feared she would act in a self-undisciplined manner in these places. As a result, Miriam stopped fearing experiencing lapses, and when they did happen she was able to learn from them.

Take the horror out of relapse

A person may have developed a rational belief about experiencing a lapse and stopped thinking that a relapse will inevitably follow any small lapse, but may still fear a relapse. If this fear is affecting her in the maintenance phase of self-discipline, then it is important that she learns to take the horror out of a relapse. She needs to learn that it is bad to experience a relapse, but hardly terrible, and that if she does relapse she can still learn from this and work her way back to greater self-discipline. The best way of learning this is for her to practise this belief while experiencing a controlled relapse (see below).

This is what Miriam did. When she felt ready and saw that it was a challenge to her, but not overwhelming for her, she practised taking the horror out of experiencing a relapse while reverting to acting in a self-undisciplined way for a week, after which she reinstated her self-discipline skills. This helped her to take the horror out of experiencing a relapse.

Having addressed both issues that underpinned her fear, Miriam was able to learn from her lapses and now successfully maintains her weight.

Please be aware that a controlled relapse and subsequent return to self-discipline is not recommended for everyone, and especially not when you may be endangering your health and well-being by having a relapse, as with hard drugs, binge drinking and other alcohol problems, and gambling.

Having said that, if you overcome your fear of relapse, this does not mean that you are more likely to experience one. It may even mean that you are less likely to experience one. For if you do not fear relapsing, it means that you are not preoccupied with relapse and therefore you can adopt a fearless approach to maintaining self-discipline. By contrast, if you fear relapsing you are preoccupied with relapse and this fear may interfere with you maintaining self-discipline.

Ellen: an example of relapse prevention in action

In this section, I will provide you with an example of how Ellen, whom we met earlier in the book, used relapse prevention in her own life.

You may recall that Ellen's self-discipline goal was to eat three good meals a day and not to eat between meals. Her self-monitoring form indicated two patterns. First, when she is alone in her kitchen she eats savoury food, and second, when she is with her partner she eats sweet food. Further assessment revealed that she eats when:

- she is bored and she holds the belief that she needs cheering up (eating savoury food cheers her up);
- she feels empty and she holds the belief that she can't stand this feeling (eating savoury food gets rid of her empty feeling);

- she wants the taste of chocolate and she believes that it would be terrible not to have what she wants (this belief leads her to eat sweet food);
- she wants to maintain a sense of being sociable with another person (most often her partner) who is eating sweets, and she believes that she has to be sociable (this belief also leads her to eat sweet food).

Ellen achieved her goals in the first place:
- by challenging the rigid beliefs that she must not experience boredom and emptiness, and by tolerating feelings of boredom and emptiness without eating savoury food to get rid of these feelings;
- by challenging the rigid belief that she must have what she wants when she wants it (i.e. the taste of chocolate and other sweet foods) and by living with the sense of deprivation when she refrains from eating her desired food;
- by challenging the rigid idea that she must be sociable and eat food when others are eating, and by refraining from eating when others eat, but being sociable nonetheless.

Ellen's vulnerability factors

When she came to plan for relapse prevention, Ellen identified the following vulnerability factors:

- being pressured by people to eat between meals when they are eating;
- feeling obliged to eat when others have made food for her when she visits them, despite asking them not to.

How Ellen dealt with her vulnerability factors

Using the principles of relapse prevention outlined above, this is how Ellen dealt with her vulnerability factors.

Being pressured by people to eat between meals when they are eating

- Ellen identified a typical example of when she was vulnerable to being pressured by others to eat between meals. She would be out with a couple of friends for coffee and one of them would buy the three of them cakes. She recognized that if she ate one she would be acting on the belief that she had to avoid uncomfortable feelings of discord.
- She pictured herself challenging this belief and holding on to the new belief that she doesn't have to avoid uncomfortable feelings of discord. She reminded herself that such feelings are tolerable and worth tolerating if it means maintaining self-discipline. While

picturing herself holding on to these beliefs, she visualized herself saying 'no' to her friend's offer of a cake and pictured herself asserting herself, explaining that she was not eating between meals and asking for her friends' future cooperation.
- She then put these healthy beliefs and constructive behaviour into practice in a number of situations, with excellent results.

Once Ellen had explained to her circle of friends that she was maintaining self-discipline, most of them cooperated with her and did not pressure her, but two friends attempted to sabotage her. Ellen dealt with these two people first by assertion, then by confrontation (see Chapter 11), and in one case she chose to terminate her friendship with one of these people, who continually attempted to sabotage her despite all of her efforts to dissuade him.

Feeling obliged to eat when others have made food for her when she visits them, despite her having asked them not to

- Ellen identified a typical example of when she was vulnerable to eating between meals. She imagined that she had asked one of her aunts not to make anything for her when she visited her for tea, but Aunt Jane had ignored her request and gone to great lengths to put on a fine spread.
- Ellen recognized that if she were to eat one or more of the fine cakes that Aunt Jane had baked especially for the occasion, she would do so because she held the belief that she must not hurt her aunt's feelings and that she would be a bad person if she did.
- She pictured herself challenging this belief and developing the alternative rational belief that while she would not like to hurt her aunt's feelings, she was not exempt from doing so and she would not be a bad person for doing so, just a fallible human being who is putting her own healthy interests first. Holding on to this belief, she pictured herself saying 'no' to all her aunt's entreaties 'to have just one cake – after all, I went to a great deal of trouble in making them just for you' and tolerating the discomfort she would feel holding her ground. While doing so, she pictured herself feeling uncomfortable; she did not feel guilty in this image.
- She then put all this into practice. She visited Aunt Jane, told her firmly not to make her any cakes or sandwiches and that she would just have a cup of tea, knowing that her aunt would take no notice of her. She rehearsed her rational beliefs in the train on her way to visit her aunt and again while Aunt Jane was preparing the tea. True to form, her aunt had disregarded Ellen's wishes and made a great spread, but Ellen declined firmly, repeatedly but politely her aunt's emotional blackmail while rehearsing her rational beliefs as she did so.

Ellen then practised such rational thinking and polite assertion whenever someone disregarded her requests not to give her any food between meals. Doing so helped her to maintain her self-discipline by refraining from eating between meals.

Balance and moderation

Being self-disciplined is not an end in itself; rather, it is a means to an end. That end usually involves you living a healthy and happy existence. Thus, people who are self-disciplined in their lives are probably healthier and happier than those who lack self-discipline.

One important aspect of being self-disciplined is that it can allow you to enjoy behaviour that taken to an extreme characterizes lack of self-discipline. Thus, if you are following a low calorie diet and doing so with self-discipline, this does not preclude you from occasionally and intentionally eating high calorie food. It does not even preclude you from having a break from self-discipline, for example when you go on holiday and eat higher calorie foods than you would if you were at home. Indeed, some people regard going on holiday as a break not only from everyday living but from self-disciplined living. Of course, you will want to reinstitute your self-disciplined behaviour on your return. My point is that being self-disciplined can be integrated flexibly into your life: it does not have to become your life! I also made this point in Chapter 3.

There are, of course, exceptions to the balanced and 'in moderation' approach to self-discipline. Thus, you will probably not want to use heroin flexibly, and some of you would prefer to abstain from alcohol rather than use it in moderation. That's fine. My point, and it will be my closing one, is that being self-disciplined in life is meant to enhance your life, not to detract from it. With this said, let me close by wishing you well in the pursuit and maintenance of self-discipline in your own life.

Appendices

Appendix 1
Setting goals for self-discipline

1 In which area of my life do I want to be more disciplined?

2 Do I really want to be disciplined in this area or am I only saying so to please others or get them 'off my back'?

3 Why do I want to be disciplined in this area?

4 Which values underpin my reasons and how important are these values in my life, on a scale from 0 = no importance to 10 = great importance?

(a)   =

(b)   =

(c)   =

(d)   =

5 How committed am I to working to develop and maintain self-discipline in this area, on a scale from 0 = no commitment to 10 = full commitment?

Commitment =

Appendix 2
Monitoring the presence of your self-undisciplined behaviour

Date	Time	Situation	Alone/with others	Description of self-undisciplined behaviour

Appendix 3

Monitoring the absence of self-disciplined behaviour

Date	Time	Planned self-disciplined behaviour	Planned situation	What I actually did	Situation	Alone/with others

Appendix 4
Self-disciplined and self-undisciplined behaviour audit forms

---

Audit of the costs of self-undisciplined behaviour:

Short-term costs to myself

Long-term costs to myself

Short-term costs to others involved

Long-term costs to others involved

Audit of the perceived advantages of self-undisciplined behaviour:

Short-term advantages to myself

Long-term advantages to myself

Short-term advantages to others involved

Long-term advantages to others involved

Audit of the advantages of self-disciplined behaviour:

Short-term advantages to myself

Long-term advantages to myself

Short-term advantages to others involved

Long-term advantages to others involved

Audit of the perceived costs of self-disciplined behaviour:

Short-term costs to myself

Long-term costs to myself

Short-term costs to others involved

Long-term costs to others involved

Appendix 5

Responding to the perceived advantages of self-undisciplined behaviour and the perceived costs of self-disciplined behaviour

---

Perceived advantages of self-undisciplined behaviour and response:

Short-term advantages to myself

•

Response:

•

Response:

Long-term advantages to myself

•

Response:

•

Response:

Short-term advantages to others involved

•

Response:

•

Response:

Long-term advantages to others involved

•

Response:

•

Response:

Perceived costs of self-disciplined behaviour and response:

Short-term costs to myself

•

Response:

•

Response:

Long-term costs to myself

•

Response:

•

Response:

Short-term costs to others involved

•

Response:

•

Response:

Long-term costs to others involved

•

Response:

•

Response:

Appendix 6
Ten steps to dealing with urges to act in self-undisciplined ways

Date: Time:
Situation:
Alone/with others:
Nature of the urge:
Strength of urge (1–10):
Purpose of the urge:

1   Acknowledge that you are experiencing an urge.

2   Acknowledge that the urge is difficult to tolerate, but that you can tolerate it and that it is worth tolerating.

3   Acknowledge that you do not have to act on your urge immediately.

4   Recognize that you have a choice: to act on the urge or not.

5   Remind yourself of the positive reasons for refraining from acting on such urges and the negative reasons for acting on them.

6   Respond to any positive reasons for acting on your urge and to any negative reasons against refraining from doing so.

7   Take purposive action even though you are experiencing the urge.

8   Ask yourself, 'Did I act on the urge or not?'

9   Ask yourself, 'If I acted on the urge, what were my true reasons for doing so?'

10 Rate immediate and later changes in the intensity of the urge (1–10).

Index

About the author

DR WINDY DRYDEN was born in London in 1950. He has worked in psychotherapy and counselling for over 30 years, and is the author or editor of over 170 books, including *How to Accept Yourself* (Sheldon Press, 1999) and *Overcoming Envy* (Sheldon Press, 2002). Dr Dryden is Professor of Psychotherapeutic Studies at Goldsmiths College, University of London.